Anxiety: A Very Short Introduction

VERY SHORT INTRODUCTIONS are for anyone wanting a stimulating and accessible way in to a new subject. They are written by experts, and have been published in more than 25 languages worldwide.

The series began in 1995 and now represents a wide variety of topics in history, philosophy, religion, science, and the humanities. The VSI library now contains more than 300 volumes – a Very Short Introduction to everything from ancient Egypt and Indian philosophy to conceptual art and cosmology – and will continue to grow in a variety of disciplines.

Very Short Introductions available now:

Available soon:

For more information visit our website
www.oup.com/vsi/

Daniel Freeman and Jason Freeman

ANXIETY

A Very Short Introduction

OXFORD
UNIVERSITY PRESS

OXFORD
UNIVERSITY PRESS

Great Clarendon Street, Oxford, OX2 6DP,
United Kingdom

Oxford University Press is a department of the University of Oxford.
It furthers the University's objective of excellence in research, scholarship,
and education by publishing worldwide. Oxford is a registered trade mark of
Oxford University Press in the UK and in certain other countries

© Daniel Freeman and Jason Freeman 2012

The moral rights of the authors have been asserted

First Edition published in 2012

1 3 5 7 9 10 8 6 4 2

British Library Cataloguing in Publication Data

Data available

Library of Congress Cataloging in Publication Data

Data available

ISBN 978-0-19-956715-7

Printed in Great Britain
on acid-free paper by
Ashford Colour Press Ltd, Gosport, Hampshire

Contents

Preface

Anxiety is one of the fundamental emotions, as central a part of what it means to be human as happiness, sadness, or anger. If you were asked to recall the last time you felt anxious, doubtless you wouldn't have to look back very far.

In its more severe forms, anxiety is also one of the most common types of psychological disorder, with millions of people around the world affected at any one time.

There's no doubting the importance of anxiety, then. But though we all experience this emotion, perhaps on a regular basis, for many of us it can seem a pretty mysterious experience. Rather like the biblical description of the wind, we recognize anxiety when it arrives but know neither where it's come from nor where it's going.

So we begin this *Very Short Introduction* by defining the meaning of anxiety. We attempt to pin down what anxiety is; what it feels like; and what its purpose might be. Though everyone feels anxious from time to time, how often we experience anxiety and how severely it affects us varies from person to person. To understand why this is, in Chapter 2 we focus on the four main theoretical perspectives on anxiety: the psychoanalytic, behavioural, cognitive, and neurobiological. We build on this discussion in Chapter 3 by considering how our genes and life experiences influence our susceptibility to anxiety.

After these theoretical explorations, we hope Chapter 4 will come as an engaging – but illuminating – diversion. In it, we present interviews specially conducted for this book with the actor, writer, and director Michael Palin and the former England football manager Graham Taylor. Each of them describes their experience of anxiety in their working lives and sets out the steps they have taken to combat it.

In the second half of the book, we switch our focus to what happens when anxiety is sufficiently severe to be considered a clinical problem. We devote a chapter to each of the six main anxiety disorders covered in psychiatric classification systems: phobia; social phobia; panic disorder; generalized anxiety disorder; obsessive-compulsive disorder; and post-traumatic stress disorder. We conclude the book by assessing the various treatment options for anxiety problems. Here the advent of highly effective cognitive behavioural therapies means that there are real grounds for optimism.

Anxiety is both absolutely normal and fascinatingly complex. It is also the focus of much cutting-edge contemporary psychological research and clinical practice. We draw on that research and practice throughout this book, but have sought to present it as clearly as possible. So we hope you'll find that this isn't just an authoritative guide to the nature of anxiety, it's an accessible and entertaining one too.

List of illustrations

Chapter 1
What is anxiety?

You know those days when you've got the mean reds...the
blues are because you're getting fat or maybe it's been
raining too long. You're sad, that's all. But the mean reds are
horrible. You're afraid and you sweat like hell, but you don't
know what you're afraid of. Except something bad is going
to happen, only you don't know what it is.

Holly Golightly in Truman Capote's *Breakfast at Tiffany's*

Anxiety doesn't ever go away. There's not suddenly a sun-lit
plateau where you're never anxious about anything – it just
takes different shapes and forms.

Michael Palin

Holly Golightly's 'mean reds' may be horrible, but they are also
absolutely normal. No one goes through life without experiencing
anxiety from time to time – perhaps before taking a flight, giving a
speech, or meeting new people. And though that anxiety-free
sun-lit plateau may sound appealing, it's probably just as well that
we won't reach it. As we'll see, anxiety isn't merely normal, it is
often essential.

On the other hand, for large – and perhaps increasing – numbers
of people, anxiety is a major problem. The poet W. H. Auden

published *The Age of Anxiety* in 1947. That now looks more like a remarkable feat of prophecy than the comment on post-war society Auden intended. The main mental health survey in the United States, for example, indicated that 18% of adults had experienced an anxiety disorder of some type in the previous 12 months. This figure refers only to anxiety that is sufficiently severe to warrant a medical diagnosis. Even so, it suggests that approximately 40 million adults in the US alone are suffering from clinical levels of anxiety – an extraordinary statistic.

A still greater number of people are struggling with levels of anxiety that don't meet the criteria for a full-blown disorder. The UK's Mental Health Foundation reported that 37% of adults felt more frightened and anxious than they had in the past. More than three-quarters of those surveyed stated that the world had become a more frightening place over the previous ten years. And almost one-third (29%) admitted that anxiety and fear had driven them to change the way they behaved, preventing them from doing things they wished they could have done.

At the other end of the scale, everyday anxiety is as natural – and beneficial – as any other emotion. We all know what it means to feel anxious; we have first-hand experience, sometimes on a regular basis. If we asked you to jot down five words to describe anxiety, doubtless you wouldn't need long to ponder.

A (very) brief history of anxiety

The English word 'anxiety' has venerable roots. Like its European cognates *angoisse* (French), *Angst* (German), *angoscia* (Italian), and *angustia* (Spanish), anxiety originates from the ancient Greek *angh*, which can be found in the ancient Greek words meaning 'to press tight', 'to strangle', 'to be weighed down with grief', and 'load', 'burden', and 'trouble'. It's easy to detect the echoes of these feelings in the generally unpleasant experience we call anxiety. *Angh* subsequently made its way into Latin terms such as *angustus, ango,* and *anxietas*, all of which carry connotations of narrowness, constriction, and discomfort – much like another Latin term that has become part of modern medical terminology: *angina*.

Ancient though the word 'anxiety' may be, it was rarely employed as a psychological or psychiatric concept before the late 19th century, and only became widespread over the course of the 20th century. Aubrey Lewis has noted that 3 academic articles on 'anxiety' were listed in *Psychological Abstracts* in 1927; 14 in 1931; 37 in 1950; and 220 in 1960.

Not that there's any evidence to suggest that the *experience* of anxiety (as opposed to the use of the term) was any less normal and widespread than it is today; it would be astounding if it were. Feelings of panic and fear, and the physical changes that often accompany them such as trembling, palpitations, and faster breathing, are regularly described in literary, religious, and medical writings throughout the centuries.

However, these sensations were seldom referred to as 'anxiety'. Moreover, they were usually explained as the product of moral or religious failings, or of organic physical defects or illness. The 18th and 19th centuries saw a huge rise in interest in 'nervous illnesses', but the symptoms of what we would today describe as anxiety were regarded as essentially physical in origin. Scientific debate focused on the question of which particular physical problem was responsible.

For example, the eminent mid-19th-century French psychiatrist Bénédict Morel (1809–73) argued that symptoms of anxiety were triggered by disease in the nervous system. The influential Hungarian ear, nose, and throat specialist Maurice Krishaber (1836–83), on the other hand, believed that anxiety was caused by cardiovascular irregularities, a problem that could be rectified by the consumption of caffeine. (Given that caffeine is now known to increase feelings of anxiety, Krishaber's recommended remedy is rather ironic.) And Moritz Benedikt (1835–1920), a professor of neurology at the University of Vienna, attributed the dizziness often experienced in panic attacks to problems in the inner ear.

The meteoric ascent of the term 'anxiety' began only with the publication in 1895 of a ground-breaking paper by Sigmund Freud (1856–1939), the founder of psychoanalysis. Under the pithy title 'On the Grounds for Detaching a Particular Syndrome from Neurasthenia under the Description "Anxiety Neurosis"', Freud argued that anxiety should be distinguished from other forms of nervous illness (or neurasthenia).

Freud, of course, wrote in German. James Strachey, who translated Freud's works into English, was acutely aware of the problems caused by rendering the German *Angst* as 'anxiety': '[*Angst* may] be translated by any one of half a dozen similarly common English words – fear, fright, alarm, and so on – and it is therefore quite unpractical to fix on some simple English term as its sole translation.' The usage, however, stuck.

The central position that the term 'anxiety' holds in psychological and psychiatric thinking today is largely a legacy of Freud's work on the topic, though Freud's theories on the matter are now largely discredited, as we'll see in Chapter 2. But other influences were at work too. One of these was the revival of interest in the mid-20th century in the work of the Danish philosopher Søren Kierkegaard (1813–55), and specifically his concept of *Angst*, an anguished dread triggered by the awareness both of our freedom to act and of our responsibility for those actions. Kierkegaard, and his thinking on *Angst*, was an important influence on prominent existentialist philosophers such as Jean-Paul Sartre (1905–80) and Martin Heidegger (1889–1976), though their idea of *Angst* was far removed from what psychologists today would define as anxiety.

Then there was the very visible epidemic of shell-shock caused by the First World War. Few indeed must have been the communities in the UK that did not include someone clearly suffering from severe psychological problems as a result of horrors endured during the conflict. (Today, these men would be diagnosed not with shell-shock but with *post-traumatic stress disorder*, which you can read more about in Chapter 10.)

Anxiety is an emotion

Theories concerning anxiety abound, but scientists agree that it is an *emotion*. Indeed, fear is usually regarded as one of the five basic emotions, alongside sadness, happiness, anger, and disgust. (As we'll see in a moment, the terms 'anxiety' and 'fear' are generally used synonymously.) By basic, we mean the first to develop in humans, usually within the first six months after birth.

This is all well and good, but what exactly do we mean by the term 'emotion'? The concept is a contested one, but there is general agreement that emotions are complex phenomena, typically affecting our thoughts, our bodies, and our behaviour. There is evidence that each of the basic emotions involves a distinct facial expression, and to some degree a different bodily (or *physiological*) reaction. When we become aware of one or more of these changes, we are feeling an emotion.

Current psychological thinking has coalesced around the idea that emotions are strong, conscious feelings triggered by our assessment – or *appraisal* – of a particular event or situation. That appraisal, which may be conscious or unconscious, determines which emotion we feel. For instance, if we sense success, we are happy. If we detect that we have been wronged or thwarted, we experience anger. And if we think that we're in danger, we feel fear.

But why do we need emotions? Wouldn't life be much more pleasant if we weren't susceptible to fear, or sadness, or disgust? In fact, without them, our lives would almost certainly be a great deal shorter. Emotions help us survive, thrive, and pass on our genes. As Paul Ekman, a leading psychologist of emotions, puts it, they have 'evolved through their adaptive value in dealing with fundamental life-tasks'. So, for example, the happiness our ancestors felt after developing a useful tool encouraged them to repeat the experience; their sadness when separated from friends and loved ones helped them preserve crucial social ties; and their anxiety helped ensure they didn't end up as some wild animal's meal.

Psychologists define emotional states in terms of how long they last. Research suggests that initial physiological reactions – which include facial expressions – generally last just a few seconds. An *emotion* lasts anywhere from seconds to hours. If it goes on for longer, it's referred to as *mood*; and if we have a tendency to react in this way, it's part of our *personality*.

Emotions are so important to us that it's unsurprising that we are often extremely successful at decoding other people's feelings. For example, research by Rainer Banse and Klaus Scherer has shown that people are adept at recognizing emotions simply by listening to someone's tone of voice rather than what is actually said. (Banse and Scherer instructed actors to pronounce a nonsensical phrase, thus preventing participants from guessing the emotion from the meaning of the words used.)

Other studies have revealed that individuals are often able to decode emotions on the basis of touch. A team of researchers in the US separated participants into pairs, and seated each pair at a table divided by a black curtain. One of the pair then attempted to convey a series of emotions – anger, disgust, fear, happiness, sadness, surprise, sympathy, embarrassment, love, envy, pride, and gratitude – purely by touching the other's arm. Those doing the touching tended to use similar techniques to communicate particular emotions: stroking to suggest love, for example, or trembling to indicate fear. And the participants guessing which emotions were being communicated were often remarkably successful in their judgements. So, if we don't know how the people around us are feeling, we may simply need to pay a little more attention to the signals they are almost inevitably sending out.

Anxiety and evolution: fight or flight

If you've detected the theories of Charles Darwin in the account of emotion we've just given, you are right. Indeed, emotions are the subject of a fascinating study by Darwin, *The Expression of the Emotions in Man and Animals*. Published in 1872, this book has long been overshadowed by Darwin's revolutionary *On the Origins of Species* (1859). But after decades of neglect, *The Expression of Emotions* has come to exert a powerful influence on scientific thinking.

Darwin sees emotions as primarily *expressive* behaviours: automatic, unconscious, and largely innate (rather than learned) physiological changes, facial expressions, and behaviours. What interests Darwin in particular is the range of actions and visible bodily changes that characterize each emotion. These actions and expressions both help the person experiencing the emotion and send signals to those around him or her. In the case of fear, Darwin notes:

> the eyes and mouth are widely opened, and the eyebrows raised. The frightened man at first stands like a statue motionless and breathless, or crouches down as if instinctively to escape observation. The heart beats quickly and violently...The skin instantly becomes pale...[and cold] perspiration exudes from it...The hairs on the skin stand erect...the mouth becomes dry...

As the title of Darwin's book makes clear, he doesn't regard emotions as a distinctly human attribute. Indeed, Darwin devotes considerable effort to highlighting the continuities (as well as

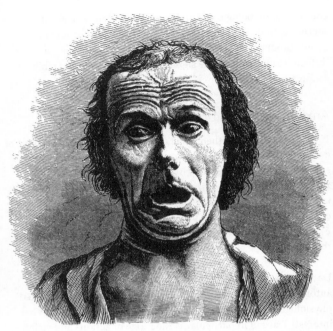

1. An illustration of 'terror' from Charles Darwin's *The Expression of the Emotions in Man and Animals*

differences) between the animal and human experience and expression of emotion. For example, he writes:

> With all or almost all animals, even with birds, terror causes the body to tremble.... With respect to the involuntary bristling of the hair [typically caused by fear], we have good reason to believe that in the case of animals, this action...serves, together with certain voluntary movements, to make them appear terrible to their enemies; and as the same involuntary and voluntary actions are performed by animals nearly related to man, we are led to believe that man has retained through inheritance a relic system, now become useless.

Equally controversially for the time, Darwin insisted that the way in which human beings expressed emotions was almost always the same, regardless of ethnicity.

So much for the expression of fear. What about anxiety's adaptive function? How exactly does it help us? The classic account was formulated in 1915 by a professor of physiology at Harvard, Walter Cannon (1871–1945). He coined the phrase 'fight or flight' to describe an animal's typical reaction to danger. Anxiety's purpose is to alert us to potential threat and to prepare us to react appropriately. And to send a signal to others that they should be on guard.

The three-systems theory of anxiety

Anxiety sets in motion a series of physiological changes, all designed to help us focus entirely on dealing with the sudden threat to our existence. These changes are associated with what is known as the autonomic nervous system (ANS), whose job is to oversee basic physiological processes – for example, breathing, temperature regulation, and blood pressure. The ANS comprises two complementary subsystems: the sympathetic nervous system (SNS), which prepares the body to respond to danger; and the parasympathetic nervous system (PNS), which controls and counterbalances the frenzied activity of the SNS.

So, for example, the sympathetic nervous system elevates our heart rate, allowing blood to reach our muscles faster (by as much as 1,200% in some instances). Our pupils dilate, relaxing the lens and allowing more light to reach the eye. The digestive system is put on hold, resulting in reduced production of saliva – hence the dry mouth we often experience when we're afraid. And new research suggests that the facial expression people typically assume when frightened – eyes wide open, nostrils flared, eyebrows raised – actually helps us see better and detect scents more efficiently: attributes that could make all the difference in dangerous situations. Without fear and anxiety, humans would surely have disappeared long ago. After all, creatures that cannot recognize danger and respond accordingly are well suited only to being someone else's prey, as the dodo would doubtless attest.

As we've seen, Darwin emphasized the way in which we express our emotions. But though this is clearly a crucial component, it doesn't tell the whole story. There is more to emotions than the configuration our facial features assume, or the way we hold our body. This is what the psychologist Peter Lang was getting at when he formulated the 'three-systems' model of anxiety. According to Lang, anxiety manifests itself in three ways:

1. What we say and how we think: for example, worrying about a problem, or voicing fear or concern.
2. How we behave: avoiding certain situations, for instance, or being constantly on guard against trouble.
3. Physical changes: for example, elevated heart beat or faster breathing, and facial expression.

These three systems are only loosely interrelated. If we want to know whether someone is anxious, we can't base our judgement simply on what they tell us about how they're feeling; they may cover up their true emotions, or even be unaware of them. Similarly, the fact that someone engages in an activity doesn't mean they're not anxious about it (just as a person might avoid doing something for any number of reasons other than fear). And it's quite possible to be anxious without feeling as if your stomach is tied in knots or that your heart is about to pound its way through your chest.

Definitions of anxiety

Bearing in mind that there is still no single definition of anxiety, let's now look at a couple of helpful attempts. The first comes from the *DSM* (the *Diagnostic and Statistical Manual of Mental Disorders*), a standard resource for mental health professionals compiled by the American Psychiatric Association. According to the *DSM*, anxiety is:

> The apprehensive anticipation of future danger or misfortune accompanied by a feeling of dysphoria or somatic feelings of tension. The focus of anticipated danger may be internal or external.

And here's a slightly less technical definition of anxiety from the US psychologist David Barlow:

> Anxiety is a *future-oriented* mood state in which one is ready or prepared to attempt to cope with upcoming negative events.... If one were to put anxiety into words, one might say, 'That terrible event could happen again and I might not be able to deal with it, but I've got to be ready to try.'

Both definitions make the point that anxiety is an emotion (though the *DSM* uses the term 'feeling' and Barlow refers to it as a 'mood state'). As we all know, anxiety is no fun; this is what the *DSM* means by 'dysphoria' (the psychological term for an unpleasant feeling). Our body may behave in unusual ways (stomach churning, eyes widening, heart racing) – hence the *DSM*'s reference to 'somatic' feelings. And at the root of it all is the perception that we may be facing serious trouble.

A closely related but slightly different concept is stress. Stress is defined as what we feel when we believe we can't cope with the demands facing us. It comprises two elements: a problem and a self-perception (specifically, that we're not able to deal with the problem in question). Like anxiety, stress is rooted in the fight or flight system. It can trigger a range of emotional responses including, very often, anxiety.

You may also be wondering how anxiety differs from fear. In fact, the two terms are often used interchangeably, and we do so in this

11

book. That said, some researchers do make a differentiation, and typically it revolves around the object of our emotion. Fear usually has a clear object – seeing a shark's fin while we're swimming, perhaps, or a dangerous piece of driving from the car alongside us on the motorway – and it often functions as a sort of emergency reaction (being mildly frightened is almost a contradiction in terms). But things are generally much less clear-cut when it comes to anxiety. Instead of situations in which we know exactly what it is that's scaring us – and when our fear will soon disappear once the threat has passed – we may not have a clue why we feel anxious. As Holly Golightly put it in *Breakfast at Tiffany's*: 'something bad is going to happen, only you don't know what it is.'

Anxiety can often be a less intense feeling than fear. It can seem vague and amorphous – and for that very reason difficult to rid ourselves of. After all, if we don't know what is making us anxious, it's difficult to know how to deal with the problem. Some experts have suggested that anxiety is the emotion we feel when we can't, or don't know how to, take action to deal with a threat. So a large dog charging towards us with its teeth bared is likely to prompt us to a fearful sprint; worries about dying are more likely to take the form of nagging anxiety than straightforward fear.

If anxiety is normal, how can we tell whether it's getting out of hand? At what point does ordinary, run-of-the-mill anxiety become a clinical problem that needs attention? Every case must be judged in its own context, but a mental health professional will consider:

- whether the individual is becoming anxious inappropriately (their anxiety is like an overly sensitive car alarm);
- whether the anxiety is based on an unrealistic or excessive perception of danger;
- how long anxiety has been affecting the person;

- how distressing it is for the individual;
- and the degree to which anxiety is interfering with the person's day-to-day life.

They'll then try to match the person's experiences to the six types of anxiety disorder – the ones categorized as such by the main psychiatric diagnostic systems – that we describe in Chapters 5 to 10.

If you're concerned about your own levels of anxiety, you'll find self-assessment questionnaires for many specific disorders in the Appendix on pp. 124–132.

Chapter 2
Theories of anxiety

As we saw in Chapter 1, the term 'anxiety' was rarely used by doctors and scientists until the 20th century. As interest in anxiety has grown, however, an increasingly rich and varied body of theoretical work devoted to understanding it has developed. In this chapter, we look at four key perspectives on anxiety, progressing from ideas that date back to the end of the 19th century to the most recent developments:

- psychoanalytic
- behavioural
- cognitive
- neurobiological

Psychoanalytic theories of anxiety

> The deeper we penetrate into the study of mental processes the more we recognize their abundance and complexity. A number of simple formulas which to begin with seemed to meet our needs have later turned out to be inadequate.... Here, where we are dealing with anxiety, you see everything in a state of flux and change.
>
> Sigmund Freud, 'Anxiety and the Instinctual Life'

An influential historical figure in the study of anxiety was the founder of psychoanalysis, Sigmund Freud (1856–1939). Freud trained as a medical doctor at the University of Vienna, specializing in neurology (the study and treatment of disorders of the nervous system). By the 1890s, Freud had come to believe that the symptoms displayed by many of his patients were the product, not of disease of the physical nervous system, but rather of their failure to deal with invisible, unconscious, and primarily sexual psychological drives. This insight became the cornerstone of psychoanalysis, which remained the predominant form of treatment for psychological problems in Europe and the United States until at least the 1970s.

Freud's interest in anxiety was marked by the publication in 1895 of his paper, 'On the Grounds for Detaching a Particular Syndrome from Neurasthenia under the Description "Anxiety Neurosis"'. As the title indicates, the principal purpose of this paper was to distinguish what Freud called 'anxiety neurosis' (*Angstneurose*) from other forms of nervous illness (or neurasthenia).

What were the symptoms of 'anxiety neurosis'? Freud listed:

- Irritability.

- Deeply engrained and distressing pessimism; the belief that disaster is just around the corner. Freud called this trait 'anxious expectation'.

- Panic attacks, often involving physical symptoms such as difficulty breathing, pains in the chest, sweating, vertigo, and trembling.

- Waking up at night in fear.

- Vertigo, in which the individual experiences 'sensations of the ground rocking, of the legs giving way and of its being impossible to stand up'.

- Phobias.

- Feelings of nausea, ravenous hunger, or diarrhoea.

- Tingling of the skin (pins and needles) or numbness.

Freud argued that, unlike other nervous illnesses, anxiety neurosis was caused by the failure to properly satisfy the build-up of sexual excitement. By way of example, Freud cited the cases of 'intentionally abstinent' men and women; men 'in a state of unconsummated excitement', for instance if they were engaged but not yet married; and women 'whose husbands suffer from ejaculatio praecox or from markedly impaired potency...[or] whose husbands practise coitus interruptus or reservatus'.

Rather ironically, given that psychoanalysis is all about the primacy of the mind, in 1895 Freud believed that anxiety was caused by *physical* factors. Sexual excitement certainly had a profound influence on the psyche, triggering the desire for sexual satisfaction, but its essence was physiological. In men, Freud argued, it consisted of 'pressure on the walls of the seminal vessels'. Freud thought an analogous process took place in the case of women, though he didn't know what this might be.

Freud's views on anxiety, however, evolved considerably over the decades. His later position is summarized in 'Anxiety and Instinctual Life', a lecture he gave in 1932. Neurotic anxiety still has its roots in sexual energy, but this energy is now seen as fundamentally psychological rather than physical.

You may have noticed the use of the term 'neurotic' here. This is because by now Freud was distinguishing between anxiety as a justified response to real danger, and so-called neurotic anxiety, which is excessive and irrational. Realistic anxiety arises from threats in the external environment; neurotic anxiety arises from within, though we are unaware of its true cause. Realistic anxiety helps us; neurotic anxiety can make our life a misery.

Key to Freud's theory of anxiety is what he called the *id*, a wild and primitive psychic reservoir of instinctive desires. The job of managing and controlling these desires, which are buried deep in our unconscious, falls to a second part of the Freudian psyche, the *ego*. When the ego fails in this unenviable task, neurotic anxiety results, and the desire is thereby repressed. Freud also suggests that our episodes of anxiety recall our first encounter with danger: the trauma of birth. Each anxious fear we experience is an echo of this fundamental event.

Freud's mature theory of anxiety is illustrated by one of his most famous case studies: that of Little Hans. Hans was a five-year-old boy who developed a fear of horses. Freud, working principally from information communicated by Hans' father, argued that Hans' horse phobia was in reality a fear of his unconscious sexual desire for his mother and the retribution from his father that he unconsciously anticipated. The 'unacceptable' fear – unacceptable because resulting from an Oedipal infatuation with his mother – is transformed into a more acceptable phobia. The neat distinction between realistic and neurotic fears is thereby overturned: Freud shows that at the root of every neurotic anxiety is the fear of an external danger (in this case punishment, possibly by means of castration, at the hands of the father).

Freud was undoubtedly one of the most influential thinkers of the 20th century, yet his ideas are now deemed more or less irrelevant by scientists. As the psychologist Stanley Rachman has written: 'The entire enterprise, including the theory of anxiety, is rich in theorizing but lacking in methodological rigour and deficient in facts.'

Behavioural theories of anxiety

Anxiety is a learned response.

O. H. Mowrer

One of the most famous experiments in the history of psychology took place in London in 1920. Directing the experiment was the then-star of Anglo-American psychology, John Broadus Watson (1878–1958). Watson was the leader of *behaviourism*, an approach

17

that would dominate academic psychology for much of the 20th century.

Behaviourism constituted a vigorous rejection of the academic psychology pioneered by Wilhelm Wundt (1832–1920) and William James (1842–1910) and of psychoanalysis, which had rapidly become the dominant approach in Europe to understanding and treating the mind and its disorders.

Behaviourism, as its name suggests, took as its subject the behaviour of humans and animals (it saw no fundamental difference between the two). Indeed, Watson argued that behaviour was the *only* appropriate subject for a genuinely scientific psychology to study. Thoughts, emotions, dreams – all were irrelevant. How could such phenomena be studied scientifically? In his 'behaviourist manifesto' of 1913, Watson had written:

> Psychology...is a purely objective experimental branch of natural science...Its theoretical goal is the prediction and control of behaviour.

For Watson and his followers, all behaviour had a simple explanation: we *learn* it. And this brings us back to that celebrated 1920 experiment. Starring opposite Watson in 1920 was an infant immortalized by Watson (together with his assistant and future wife Rosalie Rayner) as 'Albert B.'.

Albert B. was nine months old, the son of a wet nurse at London's Harriet Lane Home for Invalid Children. Watson and Rayner began by testing Albert's reactions to a range of objects, including a white rat, a rabbit, a dog, cotton wool, and burning newspapers. Albert – who, according to the psychologists, was a happy, healthy, and stoical child – appeared perfectly content with them all.

Some weeks later, Watson and Rayner showed Albert the white rat for a second time. On this occasion, as soon as Albert touched the rat, the psychologists slammed a hammer against a steel bar, producing a sudden and frighteningly loud noise. Over the next few weeks, they discovered that Albert was now afraid of the white rat, even when the steel bar wasn't struck. And not only that: the child was also scared of objects that in some way resembled the white rat, such as a rabbit or even Watson's hair.

Watson and Rayner used the term 'conditioning' to describe this process of learning to fear an unthreatening neutral object or situation because of its pairing with another more obviously frightening event. In this, they were heavily influenced by the work of the Russian scientist Ivan Pavlov (1849–1936). Pavlov famously demonstrated that, once a given stimulus (for example, a metronome) is associated with food, dogs will learn to respond to that stimulus in the same way as they react to food – by salivating – even when no food is present.

Watson and Rayner used the example of Albert B. as evidence for their theory that all fears are the result of conditioning: we learn them, usually in our childhood:

> the early home life of the child furnishes a laboratory situation for establishing conditioned emotional responses.

It is conditioning, they argued, that explains how irrational fears and phobias develop:

> It is probable that many of the phobias in psychopathology are true conditioned emotional reactions...

One baby is not, of course, a scientifically robust sample; on the other hand, most of Watson's experiments were performed on rats.

Behaviourist ideas regarding anxiety were subsequently developed by the American psychologist O. H. Mowrer (1907–82). In what has been termed the *two-stage theory* of anxiety, Mowrer argued that anxiety – and specifically the desire to avoid it – is a crucial driver of human behaviour:

> *anxiety (fear) is the conditioned form of the pain reaction*, which has the highly useful function of motivating and reinforcing behavior that tends to avoid or prevent the recurrence of the pain-producing stimulus. [Mowrer's emphasis]

Mowrer's emphasis on the motivating power of experience anticipates the *operant conditioning* theory of the Harvard psychologist Burrhus Skinner (1904–90). Skinner focused on the effect our behaviour has on the world around us. If the effect is positive, we learn to repeat the behaviour; a negative effect teaches us to try something different next time. So, for example, because we know how much pain an angry pitbull could inflict upon us, and the terror we'd feel as it rushed towards us, we're careful not to make any sudden or threatening movements when we walk past one.

Such behaviour is eminently sensible when it comes to genuine risks. But Mowrer's theory also helps explain how irrational anxieties can take hold. A person who avoids flying because of the anxiety it triggers in them deprives themselves of the opportunity to discover that their fears are exaggerated: the chances of being killed or injured in a plane crash are minute and the fear that seems overwhelming eventually dissipates. By avoiding such situations, our anxiety merely tightens its grip.

Behaviourist approaches to anxiety struggled to supply satisfactory answers to several important questions. For example, why is it that of the many people who experience a frightening experience – a car crash, for example – only some go on to develop a phobia that means they are fearful of travelling by car again? Why do many people develop phobias of situations in which they have never been? And if, according to classical conditioning theory, we can learn to be frightened of *any* neutral stimulus, why is it that some fears are much more common than others? Why are so many people afraid of heights and animals and so few scared of trees or chocolate?

More recent research has suggested explanations for at least some of these conundrums. It's clear, for example, that we do not actually have to experience an event ourselves to become afraid of its repetition. We can learn to fear from how others behave and from what they tell us. So if a parent has a phobia, there is an above-average chance of their child developing it too. And some fears may have been hard-wired by evolution. Thus, although we may never have encountered a snake or a dangerous spider, our ancestors would have had ample experience of their potential danger. The very common fears of heights can be understood in the same way. These apparently vestigial fears, relics of human pre-history, are termed 'prepared' fears by psychologists.

Behaviourism doesn't provide a complete explanation of anxiety (it would be remarkable if it did!). But its contribution has been huge. Many fears are indeed learned, if not in the relatively crude fashion of classical conditioning. Indeed, the capacity to learn from experience and formulate plans to avoid future danger is surely part of the explanation for humanity's success. As Mowrer wrote:

> the fact that the forward-thinking, anxiety-arousing propensity
> of the human mind is more highly developed than it is in
> lower animals probably accounts for many of man's unique
> accomplishments.

Behaviourism has also informed some of the most successful strategies for treating anxiety problems. The South African psychologist Joseph Wolpe (1915–97), for example, developed *behavioural desensitization* to tackle fears and phobias. This technique, which involves gradually exposing individuals to the situation they fear – for example, heights or snakes – so they can learn that there's actually nothing to be afraid of, is still the standard treatment for phobias.

And the legacy of behaviourism can be seen in today's most widespread form of psychological therapy, cognitive behaviour therapy, or CBT. At the root of CBT is the insight that unhelpful thoughts, feelings, and behaviour are not innate but learned. And because they are not innate, they can be unlearned – and often surprisingly quickly with the help of a therapist.

Cognitive theories of anxiety

> The fundamental idea is that emotions are experienced as a result of the way in which events are interpreted or appraised. It is the meaning of events that triggers emotions rather than the events themselves. The particular appraisal made will depend on the context in which an event occurs, the mood the person is in at the time it occurs, and the person's past experiences.
>
> Paul Salkovskis

Behaviourism – with its exclusive focus on those aspects of human life that could be studied in the laboratory – dominated academic psychology in the US and UK for much of the 20th century. But things began to change in 1956 with the advent of the so-called 'cognitive revolution'. Cognitivism aimed to identify and understand the basic processes underlying how human beings think; behaviourism had declined to study thoughts because they aren't the sort of thing you can observe directly.

The new approach was summarized in the ground-breaking *Cognitive Psychology*, published by Ulric Neisser (1928–2012) in 1967. Its subject was:

> all the processes by which the sensory input is transformed, reduced, elaborated, stored, recovered, and used … Such terms as sensation, perception, imagery, retention, recall, problem-solving, and thinking, among many others, refer to hypothetical stages or aspects of cognition.

To clarify these processes, cognitive psychologists mapped them out using a metaphor drawn from another boom area of the time: computing. Sensory information was depicted as being received by the brain and then processed via a series of binary yes/no steps, just like the flow diagrams on which many computer programs are based. Today, the models are more sophisticated: rather than a linear flow chart, in which a specified part of the brain deals with inputs one at a time, multiple mental processes occur simultaneously and in tandem across a complex, multi-layered 'neural network'.

Cognitivism is now the dominant strand in contemporary psychology. So what does it have to tell us about anxiety?

Perhaps its key insight is that anxiety – like other emotions – arises from our *appraisal* of a situation. Initially that appraisal, or interpretation, may not be a conscious process; often, it's a case of 'intuition'. Our senses function as an early warning system, picking up on something potentially important and then passing it on to the more rational, deliberative part of our brains to consider. When we detect a threat we're not confident we can handle, we feel anxiety. These latter, conscious thoughts about threat are crucial, and they're what modern psychological treatments for severe anxiety set about changing.

Imagine, for example, that you are woken in the early hours of the morning by a noise downstairs. How you interpret that noise will determine your emotional response. If you decide it's your cat clattering around, you might feel mild irritation at being disturbed before turning over and going back to sleep. But if you believe it may be the sound of a burglar rather than your pet cat, you'll almost certainly be gripped by anxiety and lie awake wondering whether you ought to investigate. It's not the event that determines our emotional state, but rather the way in which we make sense of that event.

The perceived threat can be either external – like the noise in the night – or internal. For example, panic attacks are very often triggered by the mistaken belief that odd but otherwise normal physical sensations – a tightness in the chest, perhaps, or a twinge in an arm – are symptoms of serious illness, such as a heart attack. Indeed, a vicious cycle can be triggered in which the physical manifestations of anxiety (for example, breathlessness, racing heart beat, queasiness) are taken as confirmation of impending collapse or death, which in turn leads to more anxiety. Again, it is the individual's appraisal of these internal signals that is crucial. This means that if you change your thinking, you can change your emotion.

But why is it that one person interprets a little breathlessness after running up stairs as a sign of imminent death, and another scarcely notices it? Why does one person assume a noise in the night is nothing to worry about, and another find themselves paralysed by anxiety? The answer lies in our preconceptions, ideas, and habitual thought processes – what the founder of cognitive behaviour therapy Aaron T. Beck termed 'schematic beliefs'. These schematic beliefs are forged through our life experiences. And they're so ingrained and automatic that we're usually unaware of their existence.

There's nothing inherently negative about cognitive schemas: they allow us to quickly orient ourselves to the situations in which we find ourselves. But Beck discovered that people with anxiety disorders typically possess unhelpful schematic beliefs about themselves, the world around them, and the future (what's known as the *cognitive triad*). For example:

- 'It's always wisest to assume the worst.'
- 'Trouble can strike at any moment; I must always be ready.'
- 'I'm a vulnerable person.'
- 'I must be in control.'

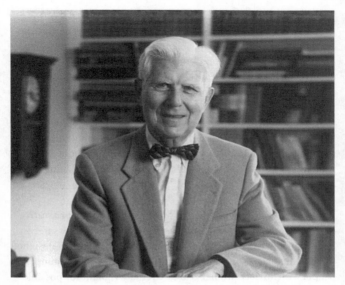

2. Aaron T. Beck is recognized as the father of cognitive behaviour therapy, the most effective form of treatment for anxiety problems. One of the world's leading researchers into psychological disorders, he is Professor Emeritus of Psychiatry at the University of Pennsylvania and founder of the Beck Institute for Cognitive Behavior Therapy. Beck has been acclaimed by the American Psychological Association as 'one of the five most influential psychotherapists of all time'

If we believe such things, we're likely to overestimate the threat facing us, and underestimate our capacity to cope with it.

Anxiety problems, if untreated, can be extremely persistent. But why is this? Anxious people can spend huge amounts of time worrying about events that have never happened to them, and indeed are very unlikely to occur. Why don't they realize that their anxiety is misplaced? Why don't they learn from experience?

This is a question that has received a great deal of attention from clinical cognitive psychologists. One of their key discoveries is that people with anxiety problems adopt a range of strategies – known as *safety behaviours* – designed to prevent the occurrence of whatever it is they fear. So, for example, a person fearful about social situations will seek to avoid them; if this is impossible, they'll fall back on other techniques such as ensuring they attend with a friend, dress as unobtrusively as possible, and keep a low profile. These safety behaviours may reduce anxiety in the short term, but they prevent us discovering that our fearful thoughts are unwarranted – and thus end up strengthening our anxiety.

Researchers have built on Beck's work to identify other *cognitive biases* underlying and sustaining anxiety disorders. Like safety behaviours, patterns of thought and behaviour that seem designed to ward off anxiety only end up tightening its grip. For example, people with anxiety problems are extremely vigilant for possible threats. But because their attention is so focused on potential danger, they tend to overlook those events that don't fit this rather bleak view of the world. This in turn can lead to an overestimation of the likelihood of danger occurring (psychologists call this *threat anticipation*) and lots of false alarms – all of which only fertilizes the ground on which anxiety grows.

There's a tendency to interpret ambiguous events negatively. This is a particular problem given that so many of the situations we encounter are inherently ambiguous, usually because it's so difficult to know how other people really think and feel. A telling example of this *attentional bias* was provided by an experiment that asked participants to spell a series of homophones (words that sound identical but have different meanings), for example: die/dye, slay/sleigh, pain/pane, weak/week, and guilt/gilt. The more anxious a participant was, the greater the likelihood that they would opt for the more threatening spelling of the words.

People with anxiety disorders are also prey to unsettling or even downright alarming images, rather than thoughts. An individual with social anxiety may possess an entirely inaccurate mental image of themselves when in social situations. Rather than thinking things through rationally, they use instinctive *emotional reasoning*. David Clark, the leading cognitive psychologist of anxiety, has explained:

> It seems as though a mental model of the patient's observable, social self was laid down after an early traumatic social experience and this model is reactivated in subsequent social encounters.

This matters all the more because research suggests that images exert a much more powerful influence on emotions than do thoughts. As with the other cognitive biases, this susceptibility to mental images enables anxiety to perpetuate and intensify itself.

Neurobiological theories of anxiety

> When it comes to detecting and responding to danger, the [vertebrate] brain just hasn't changed much. In some ways we are emotional lizards.
>
> Joseph LeDoux

What happens in our brains when we feel anxiety? Until the relatively recent development of neuroimaging technology, which allows biochemical activity in the brain to be recorded and pictured, scientists could only conjecture. But remarkable advances have been made in recent years, as we'll see in a moment.

First, however, a word of caution. Neuroscience has come a long way in a short space of time. But even were we to understand exactly how our brains function – and we are still a very long way indeed from that end point – we wouldn't thereby possess a complete explanation for our experiences. For example, though scientists can now be much more certain than ever about which parts of the brain are involved in anxiety, it is understood that no emotion can be reduced merely to a set of brain events and structures. There are always other levels of explanation, including the behavioural and cognitive aspects we've discussed already in this chapter.

The way in which such levels work has been nicely captured by the neurobiologist Steven Rose:

> The language of mind and consciousness relates to the language of brains and synapses as English does to Italian; one may translate into the other, though always with some loss of cultural resonance. But we do not have to assign primacy to either.

It's the same with anxiety; scientists approach the issue from different perspectives, but none of those perspectives has priority and all are interrelated. The best theories join up the different levels, and cognitive neuroscience has begun to do that, as we'll now see.

Long before the advent of neuroimaging, scientists had suspected that the brain's *limbic system* plays a major role in the production of emotions. The limbic system in humans closely resembles that found in the first mammals around two hundred million years ago. It is part of the forebrain, a relatively recent part of the brain in evolutionary terms, and is arranged in an approximate circle around the much more ancient brainstem ('limbic' is derived from the Latin for 'border'). Its job is to make a rapid and pre-conscious appraisal of a situation in order to help determine which emotion (and therefore reaction) is appropriate.

Also located within the forebrain are two other key components of our emotional system. The *frontal lobes* of the cerebral cortex lie directly behind the eyes, and handle many of the tasks we tend to regard as quintessentially human, such as planning, decision-making, language, and conscious thought. It's the frontal lobes that consciously think through and regulate our emotional responses.

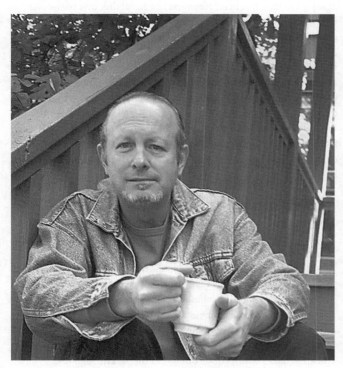

3. Joseph LeDoux (b. 1949) is a US neuroscientist and Director of New York University's Center for Neural Research. LeDoux's ground-breaking research has highlighted the central role played by the brain's amygdala in the experience of anxiety and other emotions. LeDoux is also vocalist and guitarist with The Amygdaloids, a rock band who specialize in 'songs about love and life peppered with insights drawn from research about mind and brain and mental disorders'

In this, the frontal lobes are assisted by the *hippocampus*, which helps form and store contextual memories – vital benchmarks as the frontal lobes figure out how best to react in a given situation.

Joseph LeDoux has been foremost in identifying one particular region of the limbic system as the brain's 'emotional computer', and as especially important in relation to fear and anxiety. That region is the *amygdala*, two small pieces of tissue shaped, in the view of early scientists, like almond seeds (*amygdala* is the Latin for 'almond seed'). The amygdala seems to be responsible for fear reactions in all species that have one, including reptiles and birds as well as mammals. It houses a store of *unconscious* fear memories, meaning that we can become anxious without knowing why. And it is extremely well connected to other parts of the brain. LeDoux has written:

> The amygdala is like the hub of a wheel. It receives low-level inputs from sensory-specific regions of the thalamus [another area of the forebrain], higher level information from sensory-specific [areas of the cerebral] cortex, and still higher level (sensory independent) information about the general situation from the hippocampal formation. Through such connections, the amygdala is able to process the emotional significance of individual stimuli as well as complex situations. The amygdala is, in essence, involved in the appraisal of emotional meaning.

The amygdala's connections don't end there. Through the hypothalamus, it can influence the basic processes that comprise the autonomic nervous system (for example, breathing, blood pressure, and body temperature). As we saw in Chapter 1, changes to the autonomic nervous system when we're anxious can lead to a wide range of physical effects including elevated heart rate, dilated pupils, and altered breathing.

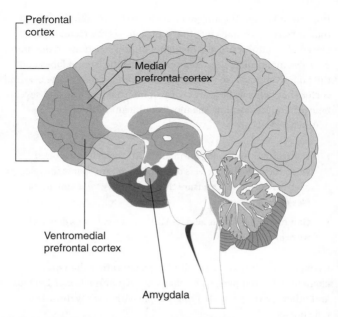

4. The brain, showing the location of the amygdala

The amygdala is able to make an appraisal of a potentially
threatening situation extremely rapidly – so rapidly, in fact, that
we may not realize why we're suddenly feeling afraid. LeDoux has
suggested that the amygdala offers a 'low road' to fear responses,
supplying a 'quick and dirty' reaction to events that is designed to
save our life first and ask questions later. The 'high road', by
contrast, involves sensory information being processed by the
frontal lobes (the part of the brain responsible for thinking things
through) *before* it reaches the amygdala. The high road is more
accurate, but slower. As you might imagine, both routes have their
advantages and disadvantages.

Important though the amygdala seems to be, we shouldn't forget that anxiety – just like any other emotion – is the result of an extremely complex process involving multiple regions of the brain. As we've mentioned, these regions include the frontal lobes and the hippocampus; also involved is the *insula*, a part of the cerebral cortex that helps us become aware of internal feelings, and several neurochemicals. Among the most significant of these neurochemicals are:

- Corticotropin-releasing hormone (CRH), which is triggered when the amygdala detects danger and in turn sparks the release of stress hormones to ensure that we're ready for action in the face of danger; and

- Gamma aminobutyric acid (GABA), which calms us down when we're anxious.

Given that anxiety is the result of a system rather than one element, what happens when that system malfunctions? LeDoux and others have speculated that people with anxiety disorders may possess:

- An overactive amygdala, and/or:
- insufficiently active frontal lobes, and/or:
- a hippocampus that doesn't pinpoint exactly which elements in a situation on the basis of past experience signal danger, meaning that they may become anxious unnecessarily.

The amygdala, as we've seen, is a kind of rapid-response unit, triggering 'just in case' fear reactions that are then appraised by the more deliberative areas of the brain. But if the frontal lobes, for example, can't make themselves heard over the noise emanating from the amygdala, we're likely to experience unnecessary anxiety over what are essentially false alarms.

There's evidence that persistent anxiety (through the effects of stress hormones) can alter the way in which the brain functions, for example, by impairing short-term memory or even shrinking the size of the hippocampus. These effects are usually reversible, but in the long term they can become permanent.

In the next chapter, we'll look at two more perspectives on anxiety. How much of a role do life experiences play in making us vulnerable to anxiety, and how significant are genetic factors?

Chapter 3
Nature or nurture?

'Murder, like talent, seems occasionally to run in families', quipped the Victorian writer G. H. Lewes. Had he been discussing anxiety, Lewes could have allowed himself a little more certainty. Anxiety really does appear to run in families. For example, a person prone to severe anxiety is likely to have a parent – and even a grandparent – with the same problem.

Why is this so? Do we inherit anxiety through our genes, or learn it from those closest to us? Are anxiety levels biologically hard-wired, or the product of life experiences (that is, our 'environment')? Over the years, both explanations have been proposed by scientists. In this chapter, we'll take a look at the evidence and try to answer that perennial question: is it nature or nurture?

The genetic perspective

Everyone is familiar with the term 'gene', and most people are aware that genes are involved in the transmission of characteristics from parent to child. Beyond this, however, we may be a little hazy! So what exactly are genes?

Every cell in our body contains 23 pairs of chromosomes, which are structures composed of deoxyribonucleic acid (DNA) and other biochemicals. One of each pair is inherited from our mother and the other from our father. Each chromosome, in every cell, contains thousands of genes – essentially extended molecules of DNA – which contain the biological rules that underlie our development. With the exception of identical twins, everyone's genetic make-up is different.

How can we tell whether genes are responsible for anxiety (or indeed anything else)? A reasonable starting point is family history. However, although this strategy may highlight a similarity between family members, it doesn't help us decide whether that similarity (or *family aggregation*) is the result of genes or environment. After all, families typically share a significant portion of both.

That said, certain types of families provide scientists with an important means of unravelling the gene/environment knot. These families are those that contain twins. Fraternal twins develop from separate eggs (hence the technical term 'dizygotic') that have been fertilized by different sperm. Like all siblings, fraternal twins share 50% of their genes. Identical (or monozygotic) twins, on the other hand, result from the fertilization by a single sperm of one egg that subsequently splits into two. As a result, their genetic make-up is exactly the same. If an anxiety disorder, for instance, is more likely to be shared by identical twins than fraternal twins, we can be fairly certain that the difference is the result of genetic factors.

Fairly certain, but not definite because identical twins may have more experiences in common than fraternal twins (although in fact the assumption that the influence of environmental factors is equal for both types of twins seems to hold). Here's where adoption studies come in. Imagine, for example, that identical twins have been separated at birth and placed with different adoptive families. (Clearly this isn't an everyday occurrence; nonetheless, it does happen, and it has been studied by behavioural geneticists.)

Each twin is brought up with adoptive siblings. Yet, despite sharing the same family environment throughout their childhood, when tested as adults, the twin and his or her adoptive siblings have very different levels of anxiety. There is, though, a significant correlation between the score of one twin and the other, despite the fact that they have never met, and between the scores of the twins and their birth parents. (Between the anxiety levels of the twins and their adoptive parents, there's no correlation.) Twin adoption studies of this type provide persuasive evidence of genetic influence, but they're difficult to run, not least because identical twins are relatively scarce.

In the case of anxiety, research indicates that genes certainly play a role. Everyone feels anxious from time to time; we'd hardly be human if we didn't. But just how frequently, how intensely, and how lastingly we become anxious is part of our personality. Psychologists call this predisposition to anxiety 'neuroticism', and we all have a greater or lesser degree of it. Heritability for neuroticism has been put at around 40%. Anxiety disorders are moderately heritable – that's to say, somewhere in the region of 20% to 40%. Research has also shown that some of the styles of thinking typical of people with anxiety problems – for example, the tendency to interpret ambiguous events as potentially dangerous or an acute sensitivity to the physiological changes triggered by anxiety – are also moderately heritable.

It's important to be clear about the meaning of the term 'heritability'. What it *doesn't* mean is that 40% of a person's level of neuroticism is necessarily the result of their genes. What it signifies is that around 40% of the *differences* in levels of neuroticism *across the population* are likely to be genetic in origin. So heritability tells us nothing about individual cases; it's relevant only to broad statistical samples. The remainder of the differences between people are the product of environmental factors.

Our genes clearly play an important role in determining our level of anxiety. But which genes are involved? The short answer is that scientists don't yet know. Several candidates have been suggested: variants in the glutamic decaroxylase 1 gene (GAD1), for example, have been associated with general emotional disorders, including anxiety problems. This is intriguing because GAD1 is involved in the production and transmission of gamma aminobutyric acid (GABA), which, as we saw in Chapter 2, helps calm us down when we're anxious. If GAD1 isn't functioning correctly, then neither will GABA, leading to exaggeratedly high levels of anxiety.

The best genetic research on anxiety looks for a gene that, like GAD1, could lead to a physiological hypersensitivity to potential danger. But, despite many exciting leads, no single 'anxiety' gene has been convincingly identified. To be meaningful, genetic studies require large numbers of people to be tested, huge amounts of research effort, and significant amounts of funding. Unsurprisingly, therefore, they are few and far between. And the findings from genetic studies are notoriously difficult to replicate: all too frequently, one research team will identify a plausible candidate gene only for subsequent studies to fail to find any link with anxiety.

Moreover, it seems unlikely that an experience as complex and varied as anxiety is the product of one or even a few isolated genes. Much more probable is the *polygenic* theory: that many different genes, each making a relatively small contribution, are involved in the generation and maintenance of anxiety. And so far the evidence suggests that what these genes are responsible for is a general tendency towards a high level of anxiety, or even general emotional arousal, rather than a specific anxiety disorder.

Identifying multiple genes involved in a complex interaction is clearly a tough assignment. But even if scientists are eventually successful, it may not be that those genes alone cause anxiety. Over the last decade or so, researchers have begun to see that there is a complex interaction of genes and environment. So, for example, although a person may be genetically susceptible to anxiety problems, they are by no means guaranteed to develop a disorder. That will happen only if the genetic vulnerability is triggered by particular life experiences. Equally, another person might experience the same events but, lacking the genetic vulnerability, will not go on to develop an anxiety disorder. As Avshalom Caspi and Terrie Moffitt have written:

> the gene–environment interaction approach assumes that environmental pathogens cause disorder, and that genes influence susceptibility to pathogens.

Let's look now at the 'environmental pathogens' involved in anxiety problems.

The environmental perspective

Important though genes are to the experience of anxiety, the environment makes an even more significant contribution. As we've seen, research indicates that genetic factors determine up to 40% of anxiety's heritability – which means that the environment accounts for 60% or more. So what are the environmental risk factors for anxiety disorders?

We know relatively little about how experiences as an adult contribute to anxiety problems (though this kind of research has been done for depression and stress). The focus instead has been on childhood experiences, and four in particular:

- trauma and other upsetting events;
- parenting style;
- attachment style;
- learning from others.

But before we look at these four factors in more detail, we should point out that none is certain to cause anxiety disorders. For example, many people endure a traumatic childhood without developing anxiety problems, and many of those who do suffer from an anxiety disorder have enjoyed a relatively happy upbringing. As we've seen in relation to genes, the process of causation is much more complex than a simple x = y. Indeed, it usually involves a complex interaction of genetic make-up and life experiences.

Trauma and other upsetting events

A plethora of research has shown that children exposed to traumatic or unpleasant experiences such as bullying or teasing, parental conflict, sexual or physical abuse, or the death of a parent are at greater risk of developing anxiety disorders.

For example, Murray Stein and colleagues surveyed 250 Canadian adults, half of whom had been diagnosed with an anxiety disorder and half (the control group) selected at random from the population of Winnipeg. They found that 15.5% of men and 33.3% of women with an anxiety disorder had suffered physical abuse as a child, compared to 8.1% of the control group. Similarly, childhood sexual abuse was much more common among women with anxiety disorders (45.1%) than women from the control group (15.4%).

Asking why these kinds of experiences result in anxiety problems might seem redundant. It's hardly surprising that children who have been beaten or sexually abused may become unusually fearful. That said, as with all genetic or environmental contributors to anxiety, there's nothing inevitable about this process. Many children suffer appalling trauma without developing anxiety disorders.

For those cases where anxiety disorders do result, psychologists have attempted to identify underlying patterns of thought and behaviour. It's been suggested, for example, that children denied the care they need can form bleak opinions of themselves and other people. The world can seem a dangerous place, and they may lack faith in their ability to cope. From a different perspective, neurobiologists have pointed out that animals exposed to prolonged stress undergo permanent changes in their brain, making them especially susceptible to anxiety. Perhaps these early life experiences bring about a similar change in children?

Parenting style

Anxiety problems aren't simply the legacy of abusive or neglectful parents. Parents who attempt to control their child's behaviour too rigidly – quite possibly because of a desire to protect them – can unwittingly send out a signal that the world is a dangerous place. They also rob the child of the chance to discover that, by and large, she can cope with the problems she encounters. (This is reminiscent of the *avoidance* strategies discussed in the previous chapter.)

When anxious and non-anxious adults are asked by psychologists to recall their childhood, the anxious individuals are more likely to describe their parents as overprotective or controlling. Memories are not always reliable, of course. However, there is some observational research with children that backs up these findings. One study, for example, asked clinically anxious and non-anxious children to solve a number of difficult puzzles. The parents were told the solutions but advised only to get involved 'if the child really needs it'. It soon became clear that parents of anxious children were much more likely to wade in than the other parents. Now if this tendency to control children's behaviour shows up in such a relatively unthreatening context, how much more pronounced is it likely to be in situations where potential risk is greater?

But though this and other studies indicate an association between overprotective or controlling parenting and children's anxiety, they don't shed much light on the question of causation. Rather than producing anxiety in children, this kind of parenting might be a response to it. The kind of research that could answer this question – assessing parents and children over a number of years rather than at a particular moment – is quite rare. But what there is points to an interaction between a child's temperament and an adult's parenting style.

For instance, one study found that it was possible to predict a toddler's level of fear by looking back to the frequency with which they had been held by their mother as a baby when they hadn't needed help. But this was only true for those children who, as babies, had been very distressed when confronted with new people or situations. Hence a parent's overprotectiveness may be a reaction to a child's innate nervousness, but one that exacerbates that nervousness – which in turn triggers even more cautious and controlling behaviour on the part of the adult.

Attachment style

An alternative perspective on parent–child relationships, and their influence on anxiety, is provided by research on *attachment style*.

Young babies tend not to be very concerned about which person is providing the care and attention they require. As you may have noticed, they're usually very happy to be passed from one adult to another, even if they have never met them before.

That all changes between the ages of seven and nine months. Gradually, the baby develops an attachment – defined by Jerome Kagan as 'an intense emotional relationship that is specific to two people, that endures over time, and in which prolonged separation from the partner is accompanied by stress and sorrow' – to one person in particular. Generally, this is the mother because she's usually the prime carer, though it could be anyone who happens to be occupying that role. The baby cries when the mother leaves (this is known as *separation anxiety*), and clings to her when unfamiliar people are nearby (so-called *stranger anxiety*).

The immensely influential child psychiatrist John Bowlby (1907–90) argued that this desire for attachment is innate: we are

41

genetically hard-wired to form these bonds because it represents our best chance of survival. Over subsequent months, the infant may develop attachments to many other figures in his/her life, but the bond with a primary caregiver – be it the mother, father, or someone else entirely – tends to remain the most significant. Bowlby believed that nothing is as important for a person's future wellbeing as these early relationships.

It is possible to get a pretty reliable sense of a child's attachment style by using the 'Strange Situation' technique devised in the 1960s by Mary Ainsworth (1913–99).

The Strange Situation begins with the researcher welcoming the baby – typically around twelve months old – and her mother to the room where the experiment is to take place. The researcher leaves and the baby is free to explore the exciting toys distributed throughout the room. A few minutes later, a stranger enters. The stranger is silent initially but after a minute or so begins chatting to the mother; the stranger then greets the child. The mother departs; three minutes later, she returns and the stranger exits. The mother leaves the baby on her own for a couple of minutes before the stranger reappears. Then the mother returns, the stranger departs, and the experiment is over.

What is crucial is the reaction of the baby to the mother's absence and return. *Securely attached* children are happy to explore the room while their mother is present, but are moderately distressed when she leaves and delighted when she returns. Children with an *anxious/resistant* attachment style stick closely to their mother, no matter how alluring the toys scattered around the room, and are distraught when she leaves. Although the anxious/resistant child will run to her mother when she returns, she will then push the mother away, or even hit her. The *anxious/avoidant* child, on the other hand, tends to ignore her mother when she's around and not be too concerned when she leaves. When the mother reappears, she'll get the same aloof treatment as before.

In a remarkable study, psychologists interviewed 172 seventeen-year-olds, all of whom had undergone the Strange Situation assessment at twelve months of age. They discovered that the babies who had displayed an anxious/resistant attachment style were more likely to have developed subsequent anxiety problems.

Why is this? Anxious/resistant behaviour often reflects a child's attempts to deal with inconsistent and unpredictable parenting, in which the kind of reception they receive depends entirely on the parent's current mood. Possibly this kind of parenting instils a sense of insecurity into the child, making them fearful that no one may come to their aid if they run into trouble. As a result, the child is constantly on the alert for danger. Perhaps too, there is a sense that the parent's behaviour is a reflection of the child's worthlessness, and by implication their inability to cope with challenges and dangers.

You may have noticed, incidentally, that anxious/avoidant children in this research were not at particular risk of later anxiety disorders. This kind of attachment is typically produced by parents who frequently ignore their child. Perhaps these children learn to manage the anxiety this kind of parenting can trigger by developing a protective independence. Unlike anxious/resistant children, who can sometimes find warmth and support from their parents, anxious/avoidant children realize that they have no choice but to look after themselves.

Learning from others

As we saw in Chapter 2, many of our fears are learned. And learned not simply from the events that happen to us directly, but from the people around us – either by what they explicitly tell us or by the way they behave. For most people, no one is more influential than their parents (though they can certainly learn from other important adults and from their peers).

A child's instinctive ability to learn from their parents was demonstrated in an experiment carried out by the psychologists Friederike Gerull and Ronald Rapee. They showed 30 toddlers a green rubber snake and then a purple rubber spider, and studied their reactions. While the toys were on display, the children's mothers were asked to react in a happy and encouraging way or in a frightened or disgusted manner.

Later, the snake and the spider were shown to the toddlers a couple more times, though on these occasions their mothers' reactions were strictly neutral. Gerull and Rapee noticed that you could predict how a child would react to the toy when they saw it again, because they mimicked the initial response of their mother. If the mother had feigned fear, the child was frightened.

On the other hand, if the mother had appeared calm and happy, the toddler reacted likewise. This may be a helpful thought for worried parents to take away. Although our children may copy our negative behaviour, they can also learn more positive messages. We can help them overcome their anxieties by maintaining an optimistic, relaxed attitude towards life's troubles in general and the situations they find scary in particular.

Chapter 4

Michael Palin and Graham Taylor: Everyday anxiety and how to cope with it

In the first three chapters of this book, we defined everyday anxiety and set out the key theories that have been developed to understand it. In Chapters 5 to 11, we'll look in detail at the major anxiety disorders and the methods used to treat them. But before we leave our discussion of everyday anxiety behind, we present two real-life accounts, interviews conducted specifically for this book. This is the sort of thing you won't find in the textbooks!

To really bring the discussion alive, we wanted to hear from figures who have had to cope with anxiety almost every day of their working lives. We chose two people who, since childhood, have been very important to us. We've long been fans of Michael Palin's work, from Monty Python and *Ripping Yarns* right through to the present day. We were fascinated to know how he coped with the nerves that we imagined must be inevitable for actors and presenters. Graham Taylor managed the football team we support, Watford FC, with unprecedented success – and no little charisma. We thought he would be ideally placed to explain how one deals with anxiety in a group of people.

With characteristic kindness, Michael and Graham each gave up their time to record interviews with us. It may seem risky to meet people you have always looked up to: fond illusions may take something of a battering. But our meetings with Michael Palin and Graham Taylor were every bit as pleasurable and instructive as we could have wished.

Anxiety as a performer

Michael Palin is an actor, writer, director, and television presenter. Born in 1943, he became famous worldwide as a member of the Monty Python team in the late 1960s. Besides his work with Python, Palin has appeared in numerous feature films and television comedies, many of which he has written and directed. He has also presented several much-loved travel documentaries, and in recent years published two bestselling volumes of diaries.

As you'll see from the following interview, Palin isn't prone to excessive anxiety in his professional life. But neither is he totally

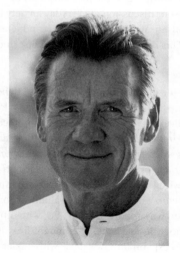

5. Michael Palin

free of it. Partly, it seems to go with the territory of performance: as he remarks to us, he's rarely met an actor who is free from nerves. Yet he can also become anxious at the thought of how other people may be perceiving him, particularly when he disagrees with the way in which he believes he is being viewed ('national treasure'), or senses that it may be critical (triggered, for instance, by a piece to camera going wrong).

Here, he is experiencing what psychologists call 'self-focus', and it can often play a big part in anxiety. When we turn our attention inwards, any worries we might have about our performance can multiply. Images of how we suspect we look to other people may pop up to plague us. Because we are preoccupied with checking how we're coming across, the panicky feelings of anxiety, and our negative thoughts, we don't notice how things are really going. Were we to look outside ourselves, we'd almost certainly discover that our anxiety is unjustified. A vicious cycle can churn into life, in which our self-focus actually causes the problems we fear (drying up in front of the camera, for instance), which in turn only increases our anxiety. As it happens, one of the techniques psychologists use to trigger self-focus in people is to point a camera at them. Almost everyone in this situation starts wondering how they are being perceived by other people. The best way to combat self-focus, as Palin has discovered, is to concentrate on the task in hand.

Palin's strategies for coping with anxiety are psychologically astute. Rather than worrying about his anxiety, he understands that what he is going through is normal and even necessary (therapists call this 'normalization'). He boosts his self-esteem, for example by reminding himself that he really can do whatever it is he's worried about. The positive thoughts and images thereby triggered (memories of a successful performance, for instance) crowd out and dampen down any negative thinking. He is a walker and a runner (physical exercise is a proven means of reducing anxiety). And he has discovered quite correctly that alcohol dampens anxiety only in the short term and is not good in the long run.

Moreover, Palin is determinedly positive, inquisitive, and purposeful: 'I think everything matters. I think that creates anxiety but in the same way it helps you deal with it because it makes you realize I'm anxious because I'm doing something that's important in its own way.' This attitude helps Palin to face tasks that he might otherwise be tempted to avoid – 'like crossing bridges on your hands and knees' – and thus prevent his anxiety really taking root (for more on the problems caused by avoiding what we fear, see p. 26). It also enables him to escape self-focus and concentrate on what he knows really matters: the task in hand.

Nervousness about performance didn't seem to be anything that worried me when I was young. The first time I performed in front of an audience for any long period of time was really in my gap year and I was in Sheffield – people didn't go very far in the gap year; I only went about four miles – and I joined one of the amateur dramatic societies in Sheffield and I could deal with that. They were quite long plays, quite a lot of words to learn. I don't remember being particularly nervous. I can't remember being particularly nervous when we did the Edinburgh revue in 1964 which decided me to take up acting. I thought: 'I really enjoy this; it's something I can do'. Even when we were doing Python it didn't seem to matter at all. It happened slightly later after Python was successful. I became a bit more self-conscious about the process.

I think for a long while you're yourself, or who you think you are. And then you become something which is somebody else's and it is their view of you. So I'd be on a programme because I'm a celebrity and I'd think: 'I'm not a celebrity – I'm me'.

Occasionally I can deal with that quite happily. You just act it. But other times it got to me and I thought 'I'm not being able to be myself'. I think that's the key to a lot of my anxiety. And the work I do is actually trying to remember who I am and what I can do rather than become a sort of figment of what people want me to be. People say: 'You're a great star; you're a national treasure; you've done all this brilliant stuff'. It just embarrasses me. It's not the way I feel about myself.

On the other hand, I think that a level of anxiety is really, really important. I've rarely known anybody who goes on stage without feeling anxious. I don't feel anxiety of the kind 'I'm a complete fraud and I'm going to get caught out one day.' I feel quite the opposite really – that I can do some really good stuff and what stops me sometimes doing it the way I want to do it is that I become slightly anxious. And yet I'm aware that I need a bit of anxiety because it's something that's quite unusual – to go in front of people, to hold court in a sense.

The main thing is that I think back to other experiences and I know that actually in the end it's making a show. I say it's just like an Edinburgh revue. I'm basically going on, got some words to learn, I've got some fellow actors, I've just got to do my stuff. So you forget really. You might speculate about the number of people who see it, but when you actually do it you know it's just like putting on a college revue or something like that. And that stuff I've done perfectly well before and I know that I can do.

So I can now really address any situation by thinking of another situation where it's been worse and I've still managed to get through. I'm fortunate because I think I'm generally positive about the world. I've not had many moments where I've had the screaming abdabs and said 'I can't do this. I want to change my job.' I've always quite enjoyed my job – whatever it is!

One has to confront these situations. If you avoid them, it's not great because there will always be that little bit in your memory, which says 'I couldn't do that; I was never able to do that'. So even if you've tried it and failed, at least you did it and it wasn't so bad, actually nobody laughed and it's been in the film and it's one of the best scenes.

On the Python shows we always used to go and have a drink before we did recordings – a little relaxant. I remember we used to go to the BBC bar and drank Ringners lager – we'd have a couple of those and it was absolutely fine. Somehow the lager sort of dealt with the adrenaline. When we were doing films like *Life of Brian*, partly because we were in Tunisia and there wasn't much drink around, but it then became acceptable not to drink if you were going to do a scene and nobody did. Ever since then I've always avoided taking drink before I perform. I'd never use alcohol to get over anxiety now because I don't think it really works in the end.

My anxiety levels seem to go up the more I'm obviously scrutinized. When we're doing the travelling for the documentaries and I'm meeting people as we go along – people think that's incredibly difficult. I don't mind that: that's fine. It's when you suddenly have: 'right, you've got to do a piece to camera'. If you get something wrong, they say 'try it again, I think you slightly hurried that bit'. And then the anxiety begins to build up.

There was one memorable bit where I had to do a piece to camera – I think it was for the Sahara series – and we'd gone to the very top of the hill in Gibraltar and you could look across and see Africa. It was the very beginning of the series and I'd written a piece about the links between Africa and Spain. And then the director said: 'Well, it's not quite what we want, can you just…' And I just thought, 'Oh God…' Well, I just couldn't get it right. When I finally did they said: 'Can we do it again because a pigeon flew into the shot and we won't be able to cut'. And then I kind of went to pieces and I just got very cross with myself.

But I don't think there are many situations where I've said 'no, I can't do that'. I've just done it and been a bit terrified – like crossing bridges on your hands and knees. But at least you've done it and you usually find that someone else around you is equally terrified, which is such an important thing in the whole business of anxiety, because if you see someone else with anxiety, not only does it make you feel you're not alone but in some cases it can make you feel slightly better: you're not as anxious as they are and so you can help them out.

For all that, anxiety doesn't ever go away. There's not suddenly a sun-lit plateau where you're never anxious about anything – it just takes different shapes and forms. If I'm going to do some acting, if I'm going to do a day's work on a documentary or something like that, I don't really sleep well the night before. I've accepted that now. There used to be a time when I felt 'God, if I don't sleep I'm not going to be able to be able to do this; I'm going to be on camera and it's just going to be awful.' And that's terrible because it's completely self-defeating.

Now I still don't sleep that well but I accept that what I'm doing is part of the process. I'm thinking it through; I'm preparing myself for the day ahead. So though you may be technically tired you're actually much better prepared. But my point is that you don't ever really free yourself of all anxiety; there's always something else you're worried about.

People see people like myself and they say 'you have the best job in the world, you're free of cares and gosh we'd all like to be like you and to be able to stand up and make a speech and all that.' I don't do any of those things without at some point feeling anxious about giving it my best and my responsibility to others. When I was young I was quite shy. I was not first in the class to put my hand up and I'd sit at the back and watch others. I like being an observer rather than being observed – which is not good for a television presenter!

I think everything matters. To me just an ordinary day matters. People say 'oh it's just a small thing, you do lots of stuff'. But you've got to do it right and do it properly, otherwise what's the point? And I think that creates anxiety but in the same way it helps you deal with it because it makes you realize I'm anxious because I'm doing something that's important in its own way.

Anxiety in managing a team

Graham Taylor is one of the most successful managers in modern English football. Born in 1944, his career as a player was curtailed by injury. He became the youngest ever fully qualified FA coach and went on to manage Lincoln City, Watford, and Aston Villa with spectacular success, leading to his appointment as England manager in 1990. Taylor is an innovator. The historian of football tactics Jonathan Wilson credits Taylor as introducing pressing into English football. He also pioneered the concept of the 'family

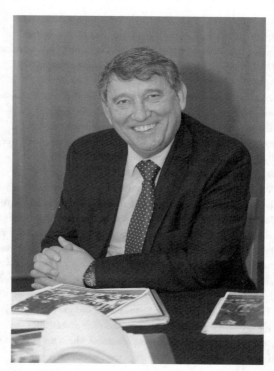

6. Graham Taylor

club', reaching out to groups who had previously felt unwelcome at football matches, and developing strong links between the club and community organizations. Resigning as England manager in 1993, Taylor returned to club management, yet again leading Watford from lower-league obscurity to the top division. He is currently chairman of Watford FC.

Taylor excelled at motivating players, often turning apparently unremarkable footballers into stars. The comment of a former Watford player is typical: 'I would have run through a brick wall for him when I was at the club and I think the supporters felt exactly the same way.' (We can certainly vouch for the truth of the latter statement.) Taylor's legendary motivational skills were based on acute sensitivity to the thoughts, feelings, and behaviour of his players. In this interview with us, Taylor focuses on one element of that psychological insight: the strategies he deployed to combat anxiety in the team.

So, for example, we see how adept Taylor was at giving his players a sense of purpose and confidence, ensuring through practice, routine, and instruction that they understood what was required of them, and, perhaps unusually, why it was required. In so doing, he taught the team to focus on the task in hand, which is the perfect way to prevent anxiety developing. Taylor took great care to get to know the players and their families, allowing him to anticipate problems before they arose. And, as he explains in the interview, he developed the ideal routine for boosting his players' confidence just before they ran out onto the pitch.

Many experiments have demonstrated that music can have a powerful effect on mood, and the success of the Watford team in 1999 provides a fascinating real-life example. The songs Taylor played in the dressing-room before games filled the players with positive feelings. They also strengthened the team spirit that undoubtedly helped produce so many victories at such a crucial time.

As we saw in Chapter 2, anxiety can be learned from other people; Taylor, full of confidence and optimism, made sure his players could not learn it from him. That said, he knew that nerves on a match day are normal. So he didn't overreact: he simply maintained the routine. And Taylor's experience as a player had taught him that people respond much more positively to praise than criticism. When working on players' technical weaknesses, he always emphasized their strengths.

We learn too how Taylor coped with his own nerves on match day: through meticulous preparation, physical exercise, and perhaps above all by focusing not on his own emotions but on those of his players. And we discover how it felt when, after years of success at club level, Taylor moved into the very different world of international management. In contrast to the iron grip in which he had held his club sides, Taylor was able to exert much less control over the England team, a situation that added an extra level of anxiety to what was already a highly pressured position.

Taylor begins his interview by recalling Watford's late charge to promotion to the Premiership in 1999, a run that saw them win nine of their final eleven games.

> We had two songs – Bryan Adams's 'Everything I Do, I Do It for You' and 'Search for the Hero' by M People – and we used to play those two before the games on the run-in. Our psychologist Ciaran, he was very, very good. There's no doubt about it: he played a part in us getting promotion. He brought the Adams song into the training ground and he said 'what we'll do, we'll get them round after training, we'll get everyone arms round one another, and we'll let them listen to this song'. So we've all got our arms round one another. I said, 'what I'm asking you is: why are you here? What are we doing all of this for?' It became very emotional – everything I do, I do for you. Those were two songs that played a big emotional part in preparing our players. They believed in it.
>
> In the 1984 Cup Final, there definitely were nerves because we were too young. Before the game, you could tell from the reaction of two players in particular. One certainly, how he was preparing, he actually sat on the floor cross-legged. Never seen it before. We had a warm-up routine for the dressing-room and he was just out of it. But looking back I made a big mistake because I announced the team after we'd beaten Arsenal. The reason I did it was that these had been the back four in the semi-final against Plymouth and I thought they needed to know. But they were too young to know and I should have kept them on tenterhooks.

How I dealt with my own nerves, I would bring the players in. I had the saying with the players, family first football second. Except on match days. Football dominates all of us on the Saturday. So what we're going to do is we report quarter to ten on Saturday morning. We would go out at Vicarage Road, not the training ground, and we'd go out at ten o'clock and in that half an hour – it was half an hour only – I took it and it was a motivational talk. We would do some sprints and all the time I was talking to them, about the opposition and a bit about what we were going to do. They go in and have a shower and then go in their cars to the hotel for the pre-match meal; yours truly runs home. And now I'm in my bath, I'm relaxed, I know I've done everything. I've finished; it's now up to you, the players.

My next bit now is quarter to three to three o'clock. In that quarter of an hour I've got to be very careful I don't say too much because I've already said it. Right at the death I would get up on the bench and I'm now taller than all of them. As they went out, I knew the people that wanted a touch from me or have me say something as they were going past. As the manager I was above them – don't worry, there's no nerves from me, fine, come on…

I'm hoping to give them all the confidence that I can feel is in me. But I've been able to get that through my running, through the adrenaline you get through physical exercise. I've prepared myself both mentally and physically, without them knowing.

Before the match, you see the players going to the toilet a lot. But that never concerned me at all. I just saw that as a matter of human nature. I've had one or two people going in to be sick. That kind of thing never worried me.

I remember being a player for Grimsby Town and the manager petrified us and on the morning of a game I didn't want to get out of bed. I was frightened and I used to say to myself if ever I become a manager whatever happens my players will not feel like this.

Getting to know the players as people, getting to know their families, was a big thing. Watford became known as the family club but people weren't always aware exactly what that meant. When I signed players, if possible, I'd like their wives or girlfriends – this was before agents – to be there and if they had family to bring their family. But the thing is of course you are signing the whole family. At one stage, we obviously had the birthdays of all of our players but we tried to get the wedding anniversaries too and then like all good managers you sent them some flowers, at the expense of the club of course! You're trying to make sure problems don't develop. By getting to know the wives and trying to keep them onside you can settle people down more because when you met the wives at the club functions they would sometimes tell you things about their husband that helped you get a better picture.

By the time of the England job, 1990, I'd been a manager for eighteen years. Walking out at Wembley, the arrogance I suppose was in me in terms of what I'd achieved, there was no fear at all. This is where I should be. This is what I've worked so hard for. I'm coming out and we're going to win.

I tended to be more nervous on the England games than I was on club games because I didn't have control. I felt it in my stomach, the feeling in the pit of your stomach that you weren't really in control of this whereas at club level you felt in control and you needed to be in control. You've got to experience a tournament before you know what international management is all about. You've only got ten games a season when you usually have 50. They're not your players, they're somebody else's players. They're not your staff, they're somebody else's staff. At that time you had no day-to-day contact with any of them at all. Mobiles were only just coming in; some of them didn't have mobile phones: how do you keep in touch with them?

There is a dislike of you by a small group of managers because you've been an opponent to them. So some managers don't want you to succeed. I'd been brought up at Scunthorpe and Scunthorpe was my side, and my second team was England. If England played everything stopped, and I took that into my managership of England – how naïve ... Every one of us England managers has come out of being very successful at club level, so you expect that to continue. I found that very difficult. What I found difficult was not being in total control of the situation. And you can't be as the England manager.

I never believed in telling a player where his weaknesses were. I believed in training and practising their strengths and it's amazing how much their weaknesses improved. If you're going to come in and say look your left foot is rank, what are you going to get? Now you can do some work on that, you can go out and say we'll do some basic things, we want to make you into a two-footed player, you'll be a better player, but your right foot is excellent, your right foot is magnificent, if you could get your left foot to be fifty per cent of that you'll be a fantastic player. Now all of a sudden your left foot can be fifty per cent weaker than your right because your manager's just told you how magnificent your right foot is and all he really wants you to do is get it half as good as that and you'll be fantastic.

Chapter 5
Phobias

Matthew is a nine-year-old boy so frightened of newspapers that he cannot bear even to see them from a distance. Sheila is a twenty-eight-year-old mother of three; she is terrified of thunder and lightning, and will do all she can to avoid experiencing them alone. Robin's fear of flying means that he will make train journeys lasting several days to avoid the misery of a few hours on a plane.

The names are fictitious, but in all other respects, these case studies are based on fact. Fears and phobias are endlessly varied, and extremely common. Think of a situation or object, and someone somewhere is probably afraid of it (you can find a comprehensive – and somewhat mind-boggling – catalogue at phobialist.com).

It's quite usual to hear people discussing their 'phobias' – by which they often mean a mild fear or dislike. But being frightened is not the same as having a phobia. So let's begin by setting out the precise, technical meaning of the term 'phobia', as defined by the American Psychiatric Association's *Diagnostic and Statistical Manual of Mental Disorders*.

What are phobias?

Here are the key symptoms a mental health professional will look for to decide whether a fear is severe enough to be termed a phobia:

- Marked and persistent fear that is excessive or unreasonable, cued by the presence or anticipation of a specific object or situation.

- Exposure to the phobic stimulus almost invariably provokes an immediate anxiety response.

- The person recognizes that the fear is excessive or unreasonable.

- The avoidance, anxious anticipation, or distress in the feared situation interferes significantly with the person's normal routine, occupational (or academic) functioning, or social activities or relationships, or there is marked distress about having the phobia.

There are literally hundreds of different phobias. But experts have identified five broad categories:

- **Animal phobias**. Among the most common animal phobias are fears of insects, snakes, rats, and dogs.

- **Natural environment phobias**. These include fears of heights, storms, and water.

- **Situational phobias**. For example, fears of flying, enclosed spaces, public transport, tunnels, bridges, elevators, and driving.

- **Blood-injection-injury phobias**. These phobias include the fear of seeing blood or an injury, or of having an injection or similar medical procedure.

- **Other types**. Everything else! Common 'other' phobias are the fear of choking or of catching an illness (as opposed to hypochondriasis, the fear of actually being ill).

Most of the several hundred phobias recorded by doctors affect a tiny number of people. (How often have you met someone who is afraid of teeth or sitting down?) A very limited number of situations or objects account for the vast majority of phobias. These are, in descending order:

- Animals
- Heights

- Blood
- Enclosed spaces
- Water
- Flying

When someone with a phobia encounters (or even anticipates encountering) the situation they fear, they usually experience a feeling of panic. This can involve some very unpleasant sensations: for example, shortness of breath, sweating, chest pains, trembling, a choking feeling, dizziness, numbness, tingling in the limbs, and nausea.

It's not uncommon for people when highly anxious, especially with panic disorder (see Chapter 7), to believe that they are about to faint, but this is an impossibility. When we're frightened, our blood pressure increases. Fainting, however, occurs when blood pressure drops dramatically.

Like most rules, though, this one has an exception. People with blood-injection-injury phobias often experience a dramatic fall in blood pressure, sometimes causing them to faint (this reaction is called a *vasovagal syncope*). No one knows for sure why this occurs, but it makes evolutionary sense. Besides fainting, an additional consequence of lowered blood pressure is reduced blood flow. If you happened to be badly wounded, this might just save your life.

How common are phobias?

Most people are prey to unreasonable or exaggerated fears at some point in their lives. Many surveys have been done on the topic, with the proportion of individuals reporting such fears typically somewhere around 50–60%.

Unsurprisingly, the number of people whose fears are sufficiently debilitating to qualify as phobias is smaller, though still substantial. The US National Comorbidity Survey Replication

(NCSR), for example, interviewed a representative national sample of over 9,000 adults from 2001 to 2003: 8.7% of those individuals had suffered from a phobia in the previous 12 months. Other surveys have produced similar results.

Phobias seem to be common in young people. A US survey of more than 10,000 teenagers found that almost 1 in 5 reported having suffered from a phobia at some point in their life.

It's uncommon to suffer from just one phobia. For instance, the NCSR's forerunner, the 1994 National Comorbidity Survey, found that, of the 22.7% of people reporting at least one phobia during their life, more than three-quarters had experienced two or more.

Most phobias begin early in life. For animal and blood-injection-injury phobias, that typically means childhood; for other phobias, onset is usually during adolescence. On average, it takes nine years for a fear to develop into a fully fledged phobia.

One striking finding is that females are more than twice as likely to suffer from phobias as males. Why is this? One theory is that men are less likely to admit they are afraid.

An experiment by Kent Pierce and Dwight Kirkpatrick provided a telling illustration of this tendency. A group of college students were asked how much they feared a number of objects and situations, including rats, mice, and rollercoaster rides.

The researchers then informed the participants that they were going to be shown a video of these objects and situations, after which they would be asked to retake the fear questionnaire. During the video, the participants' heart rate would be monitored – a procedure that the researchers implied would allow them to measure just how scared the students *really* were. Believing – erroneously, as it turned out – that their responses could be verified, the male students admitted to greater levels of fear on the second questionnaire; the women's scores remained unchanged.

Even allowing for the fact that the men in Pierce and Kirkpatrick's study tended to under-report the extent of their fears, their scores were still significantly lower than those of the women. Exactly why women are more prone to fears and phobias is unclear. There is some evidence that women are genetically more vulnerable to fear. But environmental factors doubtless play a part too. In many cultures, for example, it is less acceptable for a man to display fear than it is for a woman. So while girls may be indulged in their fears, boys are taught to overcome them.

What causes phobias?

For many years, it has been believed that we acquire our fears and phobias through a process of *conditioning*: that is, we learn them through a traumatic experience, usually in childhood. (To refresh your memory on conditioning, see pages 17–22.) Imagine, for example, that you are walking to school and a large and very aggressive dog suddenly leaps up from behind a garden fence. Fortunately, the animal is unable to escape the garden. But the incident leaves you with a deep fear of dogs; you have only to glimpse one to feel again the terror you experienced that morning long ago. Consequently, you avoid dogs at all costs – and thus fail to discover that the chances of being hurt are minimal.

Conditioning is still a useful theory. Innumerable laboratory experiments have demonstrated that it is a very effective way of inducing fear in both animals and humans (the most famous of these experiments involved Little Albert; you can read about it on p. 18). Moreover, many people with phobias do indeed trace them back to an early traumatic incident (though we might wonder whether their accounts are always accurate: in many cases, they are attempting to recall experiences from the distant past). And the psychological therapies employed to treat phobias rely heavily on insights derived from conditioning. Avoiding the situation we fear, or making a rapid exit from it, maintains and builds up our fear, so patients are helped to spend time in precisely the situations they dread (this is called *exposure therapy*). As they do so, and provided they aren't using any safety behaviours (see p. 26), their anxiety naturally diminishes. It's a remarkably effective treatment – and often a very rapid one too: just one three-hour session can eradicate a phobia that has been causing anxiety for years.

But the classical conditioning theory developed by scientists like J. B. Watson (1878–1958) comes up short in regard to certain important questions. Why, for example, do individuals often acquire phobias without undergoing any traumatic formative experience? Why is it that most of those who *do* suffer scares in childhood don't develop a phobia? (One study, for example, found that people without dog phobias were just as likely to have been attacked by dogs as those with such a phobia.) And why are some fears much more common than others? According to classical conditioning theory, any object or situation ought to be able to cause a lasting fear. How then to explain why the fear of heights is much more prevalent than the fear of travelling in a car, or why so many people are terrified of snakes and so few are frightened of electrical appliances?

In light of these questions, psychologists have rethought aspects of conditioning theory. For example, it's now understood that we don't simply learn our fears through the events we experience. We also pick up signals transmitted by the people around us. We seem to be most susceptible to these signals as children, and usually it's our parents who make the biggest impression. So if your father repeatedly tells you that dogs are dangerous, there is a fair chance that you will come to believe it.

But we don't only develop our fears on the basis of what we are told (a process known as *informational learning*). We also mimic other people's behaviour. For a good example of this *vicarious acquisition* of fear, have a look back at the experiment by Friederike Gerull and Ronald Rapee described on p. 44.

These kinds of learning may be more difficult to remember than a single dramatic and distressing event, not least because they may play out over several years. This perhaps helps explain why many individuals are unable to call to mind an explanation for their fear.

Why are some fears more prevalent than others? The answer, for some experts, lies in the concept of *biological preparedness*, summarized here by Arne Öhman and Susan Mineka:

> We are more likely to fear events and situations that provided
> threats to the survival of our ancestors, such as potentially
> deadly predators, heights, and wide open spaces, than to fear the
> most frequently encountered potentially deadly objects in our
> contemporary environment, such as weapons or motorcycles.

According to Öhman and Mineka, biological preparedness draws on a 'fear module' in the brain, centred on the amygdala. This fear module kicks in automatically and unconsciously. (For more on the role of the amygdala in anxiety, see pp. 30–32.)

In support of this idea, Mineka and Michael Cook conducted a series of experiments using laboratory-reared rhesus monkeys. The monkeys, who had never seen a snake before, displayed no fear when presented with both toy snakes and a real boa constrictor. That all changed, however, when they watched videotaped reactions of other monkeys responding fearfully to the real and artificial snakes. The lab monkeys *learned* to be afraid of snakes. On the other hand, footage which appeared to show monkeys reacting fearfully to flowers made no impression. If the lab monkeys could acquire a fear of snakes, why not a fear of flowers? The answer, according to Mineka and Cook, is that a fear of snakes is hard-wired in monkeys because of the danger they can pose. When the lab monkeys saw the other monkeys' response to the snakes, their innate fear was activated. Flowers offer no such threat and therefore trigger no prepared fear.

Perhaps our evolutionary inheritance can also be detected in the close relationship that seems to exist between particular phobias and the feeling of *disgust*. Recent research has shown that people with phobias of certain small animals – such as spiders, rats, mice, cockroaches, slugs – and some blood-injection-injury phobias are abnormally susceptible to feelings of disgust. There is a logic here. Physical disgust is designed to prevent us coming into contact with substances that could cause illness. So a fear of rats, for example, might have its roots in the animal's age-old reputation for spreading disease; a blood phobia might be based on a fear of contamination.

Conditioning clearly plays a big role in the development of fears and phobias. But, as with virtually all psychological problems, other factors are usually involved. For example, the cognitive perspective highlights the contribution of distinctive – and distinctly unhelpful – styles of thinking.

When researchers analysed the thoughts of people with a spider phobia, for instance, they unearthed some very pessimistic assumptions. Asked what they thought a spider might do if it was near them, the responses included: 'bite me', 'crawl towards my private parts', and 'crawl into my clothes'. When questioned as to their own likely reaction when encountering a spider, the participants believed they would 'feel faint', 'lose control of myself', 'scream', or 'become hysterical'. In other words, fearful thoughts play a crucial role in causing phobias.

People with phobias tend to overestimate the likelihood of coming to harm and underestimate their ability to cope with the situation they fear. They are also constantly on the look-out for any sign of the situation they dread. As Cervantes wrote: 'Fear is sharp-sighted, and can see things underground, and much more in the skies.' This threat-focused style of thinking, of course, serves only to fuel anxiety. (Incidentally, it's difficult to reconcile these findings with the *DSM*'s stipulation that 'the [phobic] person recognises that the fear is excessive or unreasonable'. On the contrary, for many individuals, their anxiety appears absolutely justified.)

The final piece in the puzzle of phobia causation comprises biological factors. Scientists believe that susceptibility to anxiety problems may be linked to an imbalance in what we might call the 'fear system' of the brain: the amygdala, the hippocampus, and the prefrontal cortex (see pp. 28–32 for more on this). That imbalance is partly genetic in origin.

One study of twins put phobia heritability at around 30% (to refresh your memory on the concept of heritability and the field of genetic epidemiology, see pp. 35–36). An analysis of male twins estimated heritability at 25–37%. A third experiment assessed how easily twins could be conditioned to fear a range of stimuli. Identical twins performed more similarly than fraternal twins, leading the researchers to conclude that the heritability of fear learning is around 35–45%.

Genetic make-up, then, is clearly part of the reason why some people develop phobias and others do not. Genes probably don't play a dominant role; the heritability figures we've quoted suggest their contribution is moderate. But without a genetic vulnerability, we are much less likely either to learn to be afraid of something, or to see that fear develop into a full-blown phobia.

Chapter 6
Social phobia

It's like a camera zooming in on a horrible, red, panicky face... I look really put-on-the-spot and nervous.

Picture of me looking guilty, nervous, anxious, embarrassed. It's my face – features distorted, intensified, big nose, weak chin, big ears, red face. Slightly awkward body posture, introverted body posture, turning in on myself. Accent more pronounced. I sound stupid, not articulate or communicating well.

See the room – big room – tables all the way round in a square, people sitting behind the tables. I am sitting at a table. Everyone else is looking at me, really staring. I look petrified – can see it in my eyes, shaking, I am talking but can't hear myself. I am leaning forward, hands in front, fiddling with my ring. The people are closer to me than they would really be.

The first of these vivid descriptions comes from a woman who fears blushing in public. Next are the words of a man who dreads being thought stupid, inarticulate, and boring. The final comment is from a woman who worries about shaking and appearing nervous in social situations.

All three individuals suffer from *social phobia*. They believe that they are not up to the task of social interaction; that they will fall short of the standards they and everyone else expects; and that they will pay a high price for their incompetence, being dismissed as foolish, inadequate, or unintelligent. In a stressful social situation, their thoughts automatically turn inwards. Rather than concentrating on the world around them, they focus on their own failings. Yet the images that spring up in their mind have little connection with reality; in fact, they are often wildly distorted and brutally unkind.

What is social phobia?

Social phobia – sometimes called social anxiety disorder – takes many forms. Some people find all social situations distressing. For others, the fear only kicks in when they have to perform a particular activity in front of others. Most often, that activity is public speaking, but social phobia can concern everything from dating to eating to using a public toilet.

These are the criteria for social phobia listed in the *Diagnostic and Statistical Manual of Mental Disorders*:

- Having a marked fear of a social situation in which the person is exposed to unfamiliar people or in which other people might judge them. The person is afraid that they will show their anxiety or do something humiliating or embarrassing.

- Almost always getting anxious in particular situations.

- Recognizing that their fears are unreasonable or exaggerated.

- Avoiding the feared situations or enduring them with distress.

- Finding it difficult to function normally because of the anxiety.

Social phobia can seem rather like shyness. The two share many features: for example, anxious thoughts about social situations; the desire to avoid those situations; and, if forced to endure them, a tendency to tremble or sweat or blush. Is social phobia simply an extreme form of shyness? Research indicates that, to some degree, this is true. When scientists compare the experiences of many highly shy and socially phobic people, they are sufficiently similar to suggest that shyness and social phobia occupy different positions on the same spectrum. On the other hand, some shy people report no fear of social situations such as parties, conversations, meetings, formal speaking, or eating in public. This implies that their form of shyness isn't simply a milder version of social phobia. So 'shyness', it seems, is a fairly broad category.

Social phobia is found worldwide, but the precise forms can vary from culture to culture. Common in Japan, for example, is the disorder *taijin kyofusho* (TKS), which translates literally as a fear of interpersonal relations. TKS and Western social phobia are alike in many respects: for example, the belief that other people will think badly of us, the feeling that we are not up to the task of social interaction, and the desire to avoid certain social situations. But there is a major difference. Rather than fearing that they will embarrass themselves, the individual with TKS primarily dreads embarrassing or offending other people. As a result, they may worry about their appearance (their facial expression, perhaps, or a supposed deformity), body odour, or an imagined tendency to stare inappropriately at others.

How common is social phobia?

Social phobia is one of the most common anxiety disorders. The US National Comorbidity Survey (NCS), for instance, estimated that 13.3% of Americans will experience it at some point during their life. The NCS's follow-up study, the National Comorbidity Survey Replication (NCSR), found that 6.8% of those questioned had suffered from social phobia in the previous twelve months. When the NCSR analysed the severity of those cases, the 6.8% figure broke down into roughly equal thirds for 'serious', 'moderate', and 'mild'. But these are relative terms: even 'mild' cases met the criteria for a clinical disorder.

Social phobia normally begins in adolescence. A major US survey found that 9% of young people aged 13–18 had experienced problems at some point in their life, with 1.3% having been severely affected. Like anxiety disorders in general, social phobia is more common in women than men (by a ratio of approximately 3:2).

What causes social phobia?

Social phobia seems to run in families, with genes believed to exert a moderate influence. Heritability has been estimated at around 40%. However, what is inherited is probably a vulnerability to anxiety in general rather than social phobia in particular.

Making a larger contribution are what scientists call non-shared environmental factors: that is, the experiences that are personal to each of us alone. What those environmental factors might be is mostly unclear. There is, though, some evidence to suggest that parents who are overly protective of their children, or who reject them, may contribute to the development of social phobia in their offspring. Certainly, it seems reasonable to assume that rejection could harm a child's self-confidence, and leave them with some unhelpful assumptions about themselves and other people. In the case of overprotective parents, it's been suggested that they may limit their children's opportunities to develop social skills.

For some theorists, social phobia is a remnant from human prehistory. Our ancestors had two options when faced with threats from within the social group: to stand up for themselves or submit. Fighting and losing could result in marginalization – or, even worse, expulsion from the group. With so much at stake, less aggressive or domineering individuals may have found it wiser simply to accept a lower social status.

What we see in social phobia today, so the theory goes, is a damaging internalization of this once useful strategy. Acutely sensitive to social rank, these individuals regard themselves as inferior. Because they are convinced that their inadequacy will be evident to all, they dread social situations. If they can't avoid such situations entirely, people with social phobia will try to be as meek and self-effacing as possible.

Does the theory stand up to scrutiny? While plausible for some cases of shyness and less severe social anxiety, it hasn't been properly tested in people with social phobia. So, for now at least, it's largely speculation.

The psychology of social phobia

When it comes to understanding the psychological processes involved in producing and maintaining the disorder, however, the picture is much clearer.

The most influential model of these processes was developed in the 1990s by the UK clinical psychologists David Clark and Adrian Wells. We'll illustrate it using a fictional case study.

Alice is a thirty-year-old copywriter in an advertising agency. She is required to give regular presentations of her work to colleagues and clients. Alice has never enjoyed this aspect of her role, but over the last couple of years her anxiety has increased to such an intensity that she wonders whether she may have to switch careers. Sure that she is going to make a fool of herself, she can't sleep the night before a presentation. Alice is tempted to avoid the situation entirely by phoning in sick. During the presentation itself, all she can think about is how awful she feels, and how ridiculous she must look to her audience. If anyone compliments her on the presentation, she presumes their praise is motivated by irony or, even worse, pity.

Let's explore Alice's social phobia using the Clark and Wells model. Although she is unaware of them, Alice has carried with her since adolescence a number of unhelpful assumptions about herself and other people. These assumptions developed after Alice had moved to a new school where she found it difficult to make friends. She desperately wants to create a good impression, but deep down – and despite all evidence to the contrary – believes she is unattractive and inarticulate.

Not only does Alice underrate her own qualities, she exaggerates those of the people she meets, presuming that they possess all the confidence and ability she feels she lacks. And she expects other people to notice – and remember – even the smallest problem in her performance. Only perfection will do.

Almost everyone experiences a degree of nervousness when giving a presentation, but Alice's unconscious assumptions mean that the situation seems much more threatening to her than it really is. She has been worrying about the presentation for days. Now the moment has arrived, the danger of making a fool of herself seems greater than ever. *Negative automatic thoughts* flood her mind: 'I can't do this. I have to get out of here. I feel sick. Everyone knows I'm a fraud.' Predictably, her anxiety skyrockets.

This anxiety manifests itself in three ways.

First are physiological symptoms: sweating, blushing, trembling, difficulty concentrating. Alice is quick to notice these bodily changes. Rather than accepting them as normal in stressful situations, she worries that her anxiety is spiralling out of control and that it will be evident to her audience – which only increases her anxiety.

Alice's worry about the physical signs of anxiety, and her acute sensitivity to them, is typical of people with social phobia. In fact, researchers have found that merely telling someone that they are undergoing an intense physiological reaction – even if it is untrue – can have a profound effect on the person's thinking. In one study, students were asked to have a conversation with a stranger. Those who were led to believe that a sensor had detected blushing, trembling, sweating, and an increase in their heart rate reported feeling more anxious, claimed to have experienced more physical signs of that anxiety, and believed that they'd made a worse impression than those who hadn't been given such information. They behaved, in other words, like people with social phobia.

Next, and crucially, Alice finds herself imagining how she must look to her audience. She sees a babbling, trembling, incoherent wreck. Not only does the image bear no relation to reality, it's so vivid that she doesn't check to see how her audience is actually responding. Instead she looks inwards for an indication of how things are going.

People with social phobia are much more likely than other people to experience images in social situations, and those images are both more negative and more likely to be from an observer's viewpoint. Research has shown that simply asking people to think of a negative rather than positive self-image leads to greater anxiety – both felt by the individual and evident to an observer. It also causes people to believe they've performed poorly in a social situation.

Finally, Alice adopts a number of *safety behaviours* – actions she believes will help her get through her ordeal (see p. 26). She overlearns her speech; quickens her presentation of it; avoids looking at her audience; and tries to think of happy times, such as her recent holiday.

But, in fact, these strategies don't help Alice. Like all safety behaviours, they prevent her from discovering that her anxiety is excessive: when she successfully makes it through to the end of the presentation, Alice credits her safety behaviours rather than her own ability to tackle a stressful task. Moreover, these behaviours – just like the self-images and physical symptoms of anxiety – pull her attention inwards and away from the task in hand, potentially hampering her performance. And they can be noticed by her audience. For all her distraction, Alice's ability to spot a quizzical look or wandering attention is razor-sharp. And when she does, her anxiety ratchets up yet another notch.

(Interestingly, the idea that people with social phobia are hypersensitive to criticism has been confirmed by neurological studies. When researchers ask individuals to read negative remarks about themselves, those with social phobia – but not those without – show significantly increased levels of activity in the amygdala, the brain's 'emotional computer' (see p. 30), and in the medial prefrontal cortex, which plays a crucial role in thinking about the self.)

Alice's anxiety doesn't diminish much at the end of her presentation. Because, just like so many people with social phobia, she endlessly mulls over her performance (Clark and Wells call this a 'postmortem'). And the more she dwells on the presentation, the worse she feels it was – and the more intensely she fears the next one.

The Clark and Wells model is often reproduced in textbooks as a sort of flow diagram. In fact, it might equally well be represented as a series of vicious circles, each of them both triggering and increasing the person's anxiety. With therapy, the cycle of social phobia can be broken. Left untreated, it can feel like being trapped within the gears of an unrelenting and remorseless machine.

Chapter 7
Panic disorder

In 1837, just a few months after returning from his epic five-year voyage around the globe on the *Beagle*, the 28-year-old Charles Darwin began to experience a number of puzzling and distressing symptoms, including palpitations, breathlessness, trembling, nausea, faintness, and sudden fear:

> I have awakened in the night being slightly unwell and felt so much afraid though my reason was laughing and told me there was nothing and tried to seize hold of objects to be frightened of.

The attacks persisted until the end of Darwin's life, 45 years later, and the scientist-adventurer rapidly became a recluse, unwilling even to leave his home unless in the company of his wife: 'I have long found it impossible to visit anywhere; the novelty and excitement would annihilate me.'

Darwin's doctors diagnosed a variety of illnesses, among them 'dyspepsia with an aggravated character', 'catarrhal dyspepsia', and 'suppressed gout'. Today, discussion in clinical journals concludes that what he may actually have been suffering from was *panic disorder*.

What is panic?

For most of us, the word 'panic' describes a sudden feeling of intense anxiety. It's what we experience when we can't find our passport at the airport, or suspect that we've deleted a crucial file on our computer.

Unpleasant though it is, this kind of experience is a distinctly 'watered-down' version of the real thing. Genuine panic means being hit by a wave of overwhelming, visceral fear, accompanied by a variety of unpleasant physical sensations, among them shortness of breath, sweating, chest pains, trembling, dizziness, numbness, tingling in the limbs, nausea, and chills and hot flushes. Heart rate may rise by more than 20 beats per minute.

Panic brings with it a range of terrifying thoughts – for example, that we're about to lose control or faint, that we're going mad, or that we're dying. Attacks develop very quickly, often peaking in as little as four or five minutes, and generally last around ten to twenty minutes.

Panic is a common feature of all anxiety disorders, and other psychological problems too (depression, for instance). In fact, one study found that fully 83% of patients with a psychological disorder reported at least one panic attack. But it takes centre stage in panic disorder, which the *Diagnostic and Statistical Manual of Mental Disorders* defines as follows:

- Recurrent, unexpected panic attacks, involving four or more of a range of sensations, including palpitations, pounding heart, sweating, trembling, breathlessness, chest pain, dizziness, and fear of dying, losing control, or going crazy.

- After an attack, one month or more of:
  - worry about the possibility of another attack, or about the meaning of the attack (for example, that it signifies a serious physical or mental illness);

- change in behaviour because of the attack (for instance, avoiding situations associated with the panic).

If you look back to the first item in this list of criteria, you'll notice the word 'unexpected'. This unexpectedness is critical in panic disorder. Someone with a height phobia might have a panic attack if asked to travel in an elevator, but the trigger for that panic will be obvious to them. In panic disorder, at least two attacks need to come out of the blue, with no obvious immediate trigger. Over time, however, the person often realizes that there are particular situations, for example supermarkets or bus journeys, in which they are more likely to panic.

Many people with panic disorder also suffer from agoraphobia. This makes sense because agoraphobia isn't in fact a fear of open spaces, but rather the fear of experiencing a panic attack in a situation in which escape is impossible and help unavailable. Because of this, agoraphobia isn't regarded these days as a distinct category of illness, but instead as secondary to panic disorder. Common situations feared by people with agoraphobia include being in a crowd or on public transport, crossing a bridge or travelling in a lift, or simply being alone – either in the home or outside it.

How common is panic disorder?

Around one in five people have experienced an unexpected panic attack, generally at times of severe stress. Panic disorder, though, is believed to affect around 2% of the population at any one time. When it comes to lifetime risk, the US National Comorbidity Survey Replication reported that 3.7% of adults had at some point experienced panic disorder, and a further 1.1% panic disorder with agoraphobia.

Panic disorder generally develops in adulthood, with surveys suggesting an average age of about 22 for onset. However, the US

National Comorbidity Survey Replication Adolescent Supplement found that 2.3% of teenagers aged 13 to 18 reported having experienced the disorder at some point.

Panic disorder is yet another anxiety disorder that is much more common in women than in men – by a ratio of two to one in this case.

What causes panic?

In 1959, the US psychiatrist Donald Klein administered imipramine, a recently developed antidepressant, to a number of patients who were probably suffering from panic disorder (though this was not a term in use in those days). Klein was not optimistic about this new treatment:

> it was more a case of our not knowing what else to do for them, and thinking that perhaps this strange new safe agent with peculiar tranquilizing powers might work.

But imipramine seemed to produce some remarkable changes in Klein's patients: within a few days, their panic attacks had disappeared. However, their general anxiety levels remained essentially unchanged. This led Klein to make a ground-breaking distinction between panic and anxiety. Panic, he argued, was a phenomenon in its own right, and not – as was then believed – simply a feature of anxiety. In so doing, Klein paved the way for the identification of panic disorder. (He also discovered that agoraphobia was rare in people who had never experienced a panic attack – another major breakthrough.)

Klein continued to investigate panic, and found that he could provoke it by dosing individuals with substances such as sodium lactate, or asking them to inhale carbon dioxide. Panic, he concluded, was a product of biological processes, and specifically a reaction to a perceived lack of breathable oxygen. (Levels of lactate in the brain rise when we cannot breathe properly: for example, if there is too much carbon dioxide, and too little oxygen, in the air.)

> We propose that many spontaneous panics occur when the brain's suffocation monitor erroneously signals a lack of useful air, thereby maladaptively triggering an evolved suffocation alarm system.

Fear of suffocation features in some panics. But over the years much of the evidence for Klein's theories has been questioned. No one, for example, has been able to identify where exactly in the body the suffocation alarm system is located. Moreover, scientists have noted that panic can be induced by a vast range of substances operating on differing aspects of human physiology – which implies that no single biological mechanism is involved. Similarly, several classes of medication can block panic attacks. And approximately 50% of people given sodium lactate, for example, do not respond by panicking: it's not an inevitable response.

Convincing demonstrations that panic attacks have a psychological component present the most serious challenge to Klein's account. For example, Ron Rapee and colleagues asked a group of people suffering from panic attacks, and another with social phobia, to inhale a mixture of carbon dioxide and oxygen. Half of the participants were not told what to expect from the inhalation; the other half were warned that they might experience sensations associated with a panic attack (for example, chest tightness, breathlessness, dizziness).

Whether or not they received an explanation made no difference to the participants with social phobia: they reacted to the gas in exactly the same way. But things were very different for the participants who suffered from panic attacks. Those who hadn't been told what to expect were much more likely to panic than those who were. Similar studies have shown that, if you simply give participants an illusion of control over the experiment – for example, by leading them to believe (erroneously) that they can reduce the supply of whichever substance is being administered – they are much less likely to panic.

Experiments like these have been crucial in the development of a *psychological* account of panic, which attaches primary importance not to physiological processes, but to thoughts. The work of David Clark has been hugely influential here. Clark argues that:

> Panic attacks result from the catastrophic misinterpretation of certain bodily sensations.

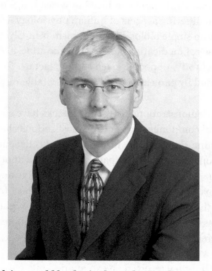

7. **David Clark is a world leader in the understanding and treatment of anxiety disorders, and a pioneer of new cognitive therapies that have transformed clinical outcomes for panic disorder, social phobia, and (with his wife Professor Anke Ehlers) post-traumatic stress disorder. Chair of Psychology at Oxford University, and Director of the Centre for Anxiety Disorders and Trauma at the Maudsley Hospital, Clark has also been a crucial figure in the UK Health Service's remarkable Improving Access to Psychological Therapies scheme**

So carbon dioxide or sodium lactate or any of the myriad alternatives used in laboratory studies don't cause panic, at least not directly. What produces panic is the 'catastrophic misinterpretation' of the physical effects produced by that substance.

Let's illustrate Clark's theory with a fictional case study:

Martin experienced his first panic attack a couple of years back. The attack seemed to Martin to have come out of the blue, though later he realized that he'd been under exceptional stress for a number of weeks because his father had been seriously ill. During that first panic attack, Martin had been convinced that he was dying of a heart attack. Although he was assured by his doctor that his heart was perfectly healthy, in the weeks and months that followed, Martin was constantly on the look-out for what he imagined were the signs of an imminent cardiac arrest: for example, his heart seeming to beat faster than normal, chest pain, or difficulty breathing. When he detected these physical changes, he became so anxious that a panic attack often followed.

In time, Martin became less concerned about the prospect of a heart attack; instead, his fear centred on the prospect of experiencing another highly distressing and unpleasant panic. In particular, he dreaded losing control of himself during a panic attack. And so Martin monitored his physical sensations just as keenly as ever; all that changed was his view of what they meant (a panic attack rather than cardiac arrest). Martin became reluctant to leave his home in case he 'humiliated' himself by experiencing a panic attack in public.

Martin's panic attacks, then, were initially triggered by mistaking normal signs of stress or anxiety for symptoms of imminent collapse and perhaps death. Later, Martin viewed these normal sensations as indications of an imminent disastrous panic attack – a misinterpretation that, ironically, helped produce the very event he feared. Incidentally, it's not only the bodily changes produced by anxiety that can trigger panic: any apparently odd sensation can do it – for example, when falling asleep, or taking physical exercise, or after having drunk too much coffee.

Like many people with panic disorder, Martin was hypersensitive to bodily changes. The psychologists Anke Ehlers and Peter Breuer demonstrated this tendency when they asked a range of volunteers, including 120 individuals with panic disorder, to silently count their heartbeat without taking their pulse. What they found was that those with panic disorder were much more accurate in their estimates than the other participants. Subsequent research has found that the same is true for children with panic problems.

Martin's reluctance to leave his home would probably be diagnosed as agoraphobia. His avoidance is actually a safety behaviour. Such behaviours figure prominently in most cases of panic disorder, just as they do in the other anxiety disorders. By staying at home, Martin denied himself the opportunity to learn that he could experience the symptoms of a panic attack without anything disastrous occurring, be it a heart attack or losing control.

Support for the catastrophic interpretation theory also comes from research into the predictors for panic attacks – that is, the factors that make people vulnerable to panic. A few years back, the psychologists Norman Schmidt, Darin Lerew, and Robert Jackson were given access to more than a thousand young people undergoing five weeks of basic military training at the United States Air Force Academy. The training is extremely tough – recruits endure punishing physical work-outs on limited sleep, are subjected to constant observation and evaluation, and, in many cases, are away from family and friends for the first time in their lives. Because of the high level of stress, it's perhaps hardly surprising that some recruits develop problems with anxiety – and with panic.

But Schmidt and colleagues found that susceptibility to panic attacks wasn't random. On the contrary, it could be predicted by looking back to how the recruits had scored on a specific psychological test they'd taken at the very start of training. This test measured *anxiety sensitivity*, which is the extent to which a person believes that the physical sensations experienced when excited or anxious (increased heart rate or breathlessness, for instance) are harmful. The higher a recruit's anxiety sensitivity rating, the more likely it was that they'd gone on to experience a panic attack.

Research like this has led some psychologists to see anxiety sensitivity as a risk factor for panic disorder. It certainly fits well with the psychological accounts of panic we've just explored: anxiety sensitivity can be seen as an underlying tendency towards the kind of 'catastrophic misinterpretation of bodily sensations' that is believed to drive panic disorder.

That tendency may be fostered by the attitudes to panic and illness we are brought up with. Research has shown that people prone to panic attacks are more likely to have witnessed their parents being highly anxious or panicking, and then misinterpreting those panics as a sign of illness (for example, by taking it especially easy or asking for special attention). They are also more likely to have lived with people suffering from chronic physical illnesses; this may make them especially sensitive to the symptoms of sickness.

If life becomes especially stressful, this vulnerability may lead to panic attacks and perhaps even panic disorder. On the other hand, it's possible that anxiety sensitivity measures not so much a vulnerability to future panic but the symptoms of *current* low-level panic.

Other risk factors have been identified. Experiencing physical or sexual abuse during childhood, for example, leads to a significantly increased risk of panic attacks in adulthood. Genetic factors play a part too, with heritability estimated at around 40%. In fact, it's been suggested that panic disorder may be the most heritable of all the anxiety disorders. Like those other disorders, however, we're nowhere near knowing exactly which genes help cause panic disorder.

Although the debate between proponents of the biological and psychological perspectives on panic continues, the weight of evidence favours the latter. Perhaps the most telling piece of this evidence is the remarkable success of psychologically based treatments for panic disorder, especially cognitive behaviour therapy. These treatments focus on changing the way people think about their physical sensations, their panics, and their ability to cope with them. If panic were primarily a biological reflex, altering patterns of thought would presumably make less therapeutic difference.

Chapter 8
Generalized anxiety disorder

When I look back on all these worries, I remember the story
of the old man who said on his deathbed that he had had a
lot of trouble in his life, most of which had never happened.

Winston Churchill

Parents in Guatemala employ an unusual technique for helping
children to overcome their worries. They give the child a small
bag containing six tiny dolls fashioned from cloth and wood.
Each night, the child tells one of the dolls a particular worry, and
then places the doll under their pillow. The doll's job is to take
on – and take away – the worry, thereby allowing the child to
sleep soundly. During the night, the parent may remove the doll.
When the child wakes up in the morning, their worry has
disappeared along with the doll.

Muñecas quitapenas – literally, 'dolls that remove worries' –
are generally given to children by their parents, but adults
use them too. And there's a reason why their use has persisted
since Mayan times: they really do seem to work. This is
because simply expressing your worries is often enough to
neutralize them. If you, or your child, are struggling with
night-time worries, you might like to make your own *muñecas
quitapenas*.

What is generalized anxiety disorder?

The term 'generalized anxiety disorder' may be new to you, but you'll certainly be familiar with the concept of worry. Here's a definition of worry:

> a chain of thoughts and images, negatively affect-laden [i.e. unpleasant emotionally] and relatively uncontrollable; it represents an attempt to engage in mental problem-solving on an issue whose outcome is uncertain but contains the possibility of one or more negative outcomes.

Despite the jargon, you'll probably recognize in this description your own experience of worry. When we worry, we become preoccupied with an aspect of our lives, trying to anticipate what might go wrong and, if it does, what consequences may follow. (This is why some psychologists have called worrying 'what if?' thinking.) While we may imagine that worrying helps us to solve our problems, this is often an illusion. Worrying is rarely constructive. Rather than improving our mood, it generally makes us feel worse. And once we start worrying, it can be difficult to stop.

A certain level of worry is normal – as the doctor and writer Lewis Thomas put it: 'We are, perhaps, uniquely among the earth's creatures, the worrying animal. We worry away our lives.' But for some people, worry can get out of hand. Virtually all the anxiety disorders we cover in this book involve a lot of worrying – as do many other types of psychological problems, particularly depression. (Technically, worry concerns problems in the future, whereas the rumination characteristic of depression focuses on past events. However, both are repetitive styles of thinking and are probably caused by the same processes.)

Moreover, worry is the cardinal characteristic of generalized anxiety disorder (GAD), which the American Psychiatric Association's *Diagnostic and Statistical Manual* defines as marked by:

- Excessive, unrealistic, and uncontrollable worry.
- Worry that has lasted for at least six months.
- At least three of the following: restlessness, feeling on edge, fatigue, difficulty concentrating, irritability, muscle tension, sleep problems.
- High levels of distress and/or major disruption to the affected person's day-to-day life.

As you'll gather from this list of symptoms, GAD can be a highly debilitating illness, with profound effects on a person's career, relationships, and overall wellbeing. As Stanley Rachman, a leading psychologist of anxiety, has written:

> Affected people go to great lengths to avoid risks, engage in repeated checking, pursue and recommend cautious behaviour, regulate their diet carefully, practice the most hygienic habits, and generally engage in overprotective behaviour. Despite all these attempts they seldom achieve a sense of safety or of contentment.

How common is GAD?

Almost everyone worries from time to time. Some of us, though, worry more often and more intensely. In one study:

- 38% of people reported worrying at least once a day. 19.4% worried once every two to three days. And 15% worried about once a month.
- For 9% of people, their spells of worrying lasted two or more hours. 11% worried for one to two hours. 18% worried for between ten and sixty minutes; 38% for one to ten minutes; and a happy 24% said they worried for less than a minute at a time.

About 3% of people suffer from generalized anxiety disorder, and women are twice as likely to be affected as men. Research indicates that around 2% of young people may have experienced GAD by the age of 18, with 0.3% severely affected.

What causes GAD?

Generalized anxiety disorder is a relatively new concept, appearing in the *Diagnostic and Statistical Manual* for the first time in 1980, and only really coming into its own as a diagnostic category in the 1990s. This partly explains why research on worry is a relatively recent development, with no single account dominant.

That said, several theories of worry have been influential, and we begin this section on the causes of GAD by discussing the four main ones.

Theories of worry

The metacognitive model

The word 'metacognitive' means the beliefs we hold about our thoughts. And the theory developed by Adrian Wells puts metacognitive beliefs about worry firmly at the centre of GAD.

Wells highlights two types of metacognitive beliefs: positive and negative. Like many people, whether they have an anxiety problem or not, individuals with GAD tend to see worry as beneficial. They may believe, for instance, that worrying helps them to anticipate and solve problems; that it provides the motivation necessary to tackle those problems; or that it prepares them for the worst if a solution can't be found. Despite realizing that it is pure superstition, they may even feel that by worrying about an event they can prevent it occurring.

Clearly, someone who thinks of worry in such positive terms may do rather a lot of it. But people with GAD, unlike other anxious individuals, also hold a number of negative views of worry: principally, that worry is uncontrollable – once you start, it's almost impossible to stop; and that worry is dangerous – as a sign of looming insanity, for example.

It's this painful combination of positive and negative views about worry that distinguishes GAD – and makes life such a misery for those who suffer from it. These people worry because they feel it's the right thing to do; and yet worrying is a source of huge distress. Indeed, as this theory has helped reveal, people with GAD even worry about worry.

The cognitive avoidance theory

Rather differently, Tom Borkovec of Penn State University argues that worry is principally an avoidance strategy. What we're avoiding is the present, and we do this when we worry by focusing on the future. Borkovec suggests that this avoidance takes three forms.

First, we worry because we believe it will help us to prevent disaster occurring or, if it does happen, to cope with it.

Next, worry about relatively superficial or unlikely threats distracts us from more distressing problems. Borkovec notes, for instance, that people with GAD report more trauma in their lives, and worse relationships.

Finally, worry suppresses feelings, allowing us to avoid the full emotional impact of a feared event. Worry, argues Borkovec, is essentially verbal thought. And verbal thought is not a good medium for emotions. To really feel something, we need to visualize it, but worry distracts us from such images. Borkovec cites research indicating that worry reduces bodily arousal (such as heart rate) in response to threatening images. He concludes:

> In sum, worriers may escape fearful imagery by focusing on the verbal channel while thinking about the future in more abstract terms, e.g. 'something awful will happen', with few concrete details.

Intolerance of uncertainty

For Naomi Koerner and Michel Dugas, GAD is founded on *intolerance of uncertainty*:

> Individuals who are intolerant of uncertainty believe that uncertainty is stressful and upsetting, that being uncertain about the future is unfair, that unexpected events are negative and should be avoided, and that uncertainty interferes with one's ability to function.

Worry, almost by definition, is an attempt to anticipate and control uncertain future events. It seems logical, then, that people with a strong intolerance of uncertainty will become persistent worriers.

Koerner and Dugas speculate that the progression from intolerance of uncertainty to worry may be influenced by three factors. First are the positive beliefs about worry we touched on when discussing the metacognitive model. Second are the forms of cognitive avoidance identified by Borkovec. And third is the belief, held by many people with GAD, that they are poor at solving problems: 'because some degree of uncertainty is inherent to most problems, it is easy to see how individuals with GAD could become frustrated and overwhelmed with solving even minor problems' – which only increases their anxiety and fuels their worry.

The mood-as-input theory

The mood-as-input theory of worry was formulated by the British psychologist Graham Davey, though it's nicely demonstrated by an experiment carried out by other researchers a few years earlier. Half of the participants in the experiment were put into a bad mood, and the other half into a good mood. Then they were each asked to come up with a list of birds' names. Half were told they could stop when they felt like it (the 'feel like continuing' stop rule) and half to continue until they could think of no more names (the 'as many as can' stop rule).

The participants' response to those stop rules depended on their mood. For the 'feel like continuing' group, those feeling upbeat persevered longer than those in a negative mood. But the situation was reversed in the 'as many as can' group: those in a bad mood were more likely to persist with the task.

Davey argues that this experiment encapsulates two essential features of severe worry. First is the fact that our sense of whether or not we've completed a task satisfactorily is often based on our mood, rather than any objective measurement. This is particularly true for tasks which don't have an obvious end point, such as worrying. A negative mood indicates that the task hasn't been completed. So someone who feels anxious or unhappy – as people suffering from GAD generally are – is likely to feel that they haven't yet worried enough.

The second point is that persistent worriers tend to use the 'as many as can' stop rule. This may be partly because there seems to be a natural tendency to opt for such a rule when we're feeling down, and partly because worriers often hold some fairly rigid beliefs: for example, that worrying is essential if disaster is to be averted; that only perfection will do; and that uncertainty is undesirable. But the 'as many as can' stop rule can be a tough one to follow. And with activities as open-ended as worry, an obvious conclusion is rarely in sight.

Biological perspectives on GAD

What do we know about what's happening in the brain when we worry? Neurological research on worry is in its early days, but some insights have already emerged.

In one study, scientists asked people with GAD and non-anxious individuals to spend time thinking about a variety of faces and sentences, some of which had no emotional resonance while others were designed to induce worry. During the task, the participants' brain activity was recorded in a functional magnetic resonance imaging (fMRI) scanner.

For both the anxious and non-anxious groups, the same areas of the brain were activated when they worried. These areas were the medial prefrontal cortex, which plays an important role in our thoughts about our self, and the anterior cingulate region, which – among other tasks – is involved in problem-solving and the processing of emotions. But there was a difference between the two groups. In the individuals with GAD, the 'worrying' areas of the brain remained active even when they were told to stop thinking about a sentence or face and instead relax. We know that people with GAD find it extremely difficult to stop worrying; this experiment provides neurological confirmation.

When it comes to genetic influences, the evidence suggests that these are less significant for GAD than for many other anxiety disorders. The disorder seems to run in families, at least to a degree, but this seems to be overwhelmingly the result of environmental factors. No genetic influence at all was found in two twin studies, while three others estimated heritability at around 20%. Moreover, the genetic vulnerability for GAD is very close indeed to that for depression, leading some researchers to suggest that 'from a genetic perspective, MD [major depression] and GAD seemed to be the same disorder'.

Social perspectives on GAD

GAD and depression may appear virtually identical in terms of genetic influence, but if we look at the long-term risk factors for each disorder, greater differences emerge.

Researchers who followed 1,000 New Zealanders from infancy to age 32 discovered that, although clinical depression and GAD share some risk factors, the differences are much more significant. Depression is linked to a family history of the illness and to problems in adolescence. GAD, on the other hand, is strongly associated with childhood experience, specifically a low socio-economic background; anxious, hostile, or abusive parenting; inhibited temperament; a tendency to worry, or to be unhappy or fearful; and behavioural problems such as bullying, fighting, stealing, tantrums, and lying.

Similarly, when psychologists interviewed a group of Dutch primary school children they found that the children who regarded their parents as anxious or rejecting reported higher levels of worry. So too did those who saw themselves as 'insecurely attached' – indicating a fundamental problem in their relationship with their parents (for more on attachment styles, see p. 41). Clearly, the researchers were relying on the children's own accounts. And it's not impossible that the children who reported difficulties in their parenting did so *because* they were prone to worry. Nevertheless, the research reinforces the link between worry and childhood experience suggested by the New Zealand study.

Chapter 9
Obsessive-compulsive disorder

Have you ever left the house and then hurried back, maybe several times, to check that you've locked the front door or turned off the cooker? Have you ever found yourself unpacking your bag yet again on the way to the airport just to be sure that you haven't forgotten your passport? And do you sometimes feel the need to wash your hands repeatedly after going to the toilet or touching something dirty?

How about strange thoughts that pop into your mind as if from nowhere? Do you ever find yourself thinking, for example, that you're about to hit someone? Or shout or swear in the most inappropriate situations – at a funeral, perhaps, or in a library?

If you've answered yes to any of these questions, don't worry. Virtually everyone experiences impulses like this occasionally. And they can sometimes seem quite bizarre. Here's a selection volunteered by members of the general public:

- Impulse to push someone in front of a train.
- Wishing a person would die.
- Thought of throwing a baby down the stairs.
- Image of being in a car accident, trapped under water.
- Thoughts of catching a disease from touching a toilet seat.
- Idea that dirt is always on my hand.

- Impulse to say something hurtful.
- Thought of blurting out something in church.
- Thoughts of 'unnatural' sexual acts.
- Idea of electrical appliances catching fire while I'm out.
- Idea of my home being broken into.
- Thought that I haven't applied my car's handbrake properly and that the car will crash into traffic while I'm away.

What is obsessive-compulsive disorder?

For a small proportion of people, these normal thoughts and urges can spiral out of control, dominating their life and developing into an extremely powerful and distressing set of worries and rituals that is termed *obsessive-compulsive disorder* (OCD).

The word 'obsession' is often used to denote a keen interest in something, but it has a specific and quite different meaning here. *Obsessions* in OCD are upsetting and unwanted thoughts, images, and impulses that constantly recur, sometimes throughout the day and night. So distressing are they that people with OCD use a variety of elaborate and time-consuming rituals to try to make them disappear, or to prevent the harm they seem to predict. These rituals are called *compulsions* and they can be actions (checking that your home is spotlessly clean, for example) or thoughts (for instance, repeating a particular 'neutralizing' phrase in your mind).

(Incidentally, the name 'obsessive-compulsive disorder' is the result of a compromise. When the German psychiatric term *Zwangvorstellung*, literally 'irresistible thoughts', was translated into English, the British opted for 'obsession' and the Americans for 'compulsion'.)

A person is likely to be diagnosed with OCD if:

- They have regular unwanted and inappropriate thoughts, impulses, or images.

- These thoughts, impulses, or images are distressing, and are not simply exaggerated worries about real-life problems.

- They try to ignore or suppress the thoughts.

- They recognize that the thoughts are the product of their own mind.

- They engage in repetitive and ritualistic actions or thoughts (i.e. compulsions) in response to their obsessions.

- The compulsions aim to reduce the distress caused by the obsessions, or prevent some dreaded event, but are excessive and unrealistic.

- They have recognized that the obsessions or compulsions are unreasonable (this recognition often comes and goes, depending on how the person is feeling).

- The obsessions or compulsions cause significant distress, take up more than an hour a day, or have a major impact on the person's normal life.

In its severest form, OCD can have a devastating effect, taking up so much of the person's time that they're unable to carry on normal life. It's not uncommon for someone with fears about contamination, for example, to spend many hours washing and showering each day. You can get a sense of the potential seriousness of OCD from the fact that it's the anxiety disorder most likely to cause hospitalization.

Sometimes there's a logical connection between a compulsion and an obsession (for example, constant washing resulting from a fear of catching a disease). In other cases, there's no obvious rhyme or reason (for example, a person might perform counting rituals to prevent their loved ones coming to harm). The vast majority of people with obsessions also have compulsions, but they can each occur independently.

OCD is a pretty heterogeneous category, encompassing a very broad range of anxieties and symptoms. In an effort to clarify that diversity, scientists have identified five 'dimensions':

Obsession	Compulsion
Inflicting harm, or failing to prevent harm	Checking; seeking reassurance
Symmetry	Ordering and counting
Contamination	Washing and cleaning
Sex, violence, religion	Various
Hoarding (obtaining and keeping items that seem to others to be of little or no value)	Collecting

Despite this effort to impose order, debate over exactly what should be classified as OCD continues. Some experts, for example, have argued that hoarding is a distinctive form of illness in its own right. Others have argued that certain religious obsessions should be regarded not as a type of OCD but as 'scrupulosity disorder'.

How common is OCD?

Intrusive thoughts, as we've seen, are normal, with around 80% of people experiencing them from time to time. It's been estimated that the average person has around 4,000 thoughts each day, most of them lasting about five seconds. Approximately 13% of these thoughts (i.e. around 500) appear in our minds spontaneously.

Roughly 2–3% of people develop OCD at some point in their life. The recent US National Comorbidity Survey Replication (NCSR) estimated that 1.2% of the people questioned had suffered from OCD over the past twelve months, with the lifetime figure put at 2.3%. The most common forms of the illness were checking, hoarding, and ordering. On average, obsessions took up 5.9 hours a day, and compulsions 4.6 hours. Given the amount of time consumed by OCD, it's hardly surprising that almost two-thirds of those who'd experienced the illness in the previous year reported that it had severely interfered with their day-to-day life.

As we've seen, many anxiety disorders seem to be much more prevalent among women than men. The picture is less clear in the case of OCD; the NCSR reported that women were at significantly greater risk than men, yet other studies have found no gender differences.

OCD can develop at any age, but most usually occurs during late adolescence or early adulthood (in the NCSR, average age for onset was 19.5 years).

What causes OCD?

Psychological perspectives

Up until the 1970s, most mental health professionals looked at OCD through the lens of psychoanalysis, which regarded obsessions as irruptions of deep, instinctive, and principally sexual urges, and compulsions as attempts to control these urges. Persuading a person with OCD to abandon their compulsions was seen as a sure-fire means to propel the individual into psychosis (the technical term for insanity).

That consensus began to change with the ground-breaking work of behavioural psychologists such as Stanley Rachman. The behaviourists argued that obsessions arise from conditioned anxiety. A person who learns to fear contamination, for instance, may become anxious at the sight or mere thought of dirt. When they wash themselves, their anxiety quickly subsides. And because washing makes them feel so much better, they'll do it again the next time they feel anxious (this is an example of *positive reinforcement*).

But Rachman and colleagues demonstrated that it isn't necessary to use compulsions to reduce the anxiety triggered by obsessions. In what's known as *exposure and response prevention* treatment, patients are taught to refrain from reacting compulsively. What they discover is that their anxiety will decrease all by itself. The debilitating cycle of obsession and compulsion is broken, and lasting improvement in OCD symptoms usually follows.

Cognitive theories of OCD have built on the insights of behaviourist approaches. The main model has been formulated by Paul Salkovskis, who argues that what distinguishes the person with OCD is not unpleasant, intrusive impulses – as we've seen, almost everyone experiences those – but rather the way they *interpret* such impulses.

At the core of that interpretation is the idea that, as Salkovskis puts it, 'the person may be, may have been, or may come to be, responsible for harm or its prevention' (either to oneself or others). So someone with OCD may believe that, if they don't constantly wash themselves or clean their home, they or their loved ones will develop a fatal illness. A person disturbed by ideas of violence may believe that such thoughts prove they are a danger to others. And an individual who sees an image of their home in flames may fear that this is what will happen unless they repeatedly check that electrical appliances have been switched off. Salkovskis argues that these feelings of responsibility are generally the result of early life experiences – for example, the attitudes with which we were brought up.

Understandably, such feelings can cause great anxiety. The person with OCD tries to rid themselves of that anxiety (and prevent the disaster they fear) through their compulsions. Unfortunately, although a compulsion may bring short-term relief, in the long run it only serves to maintain and indeed increase the anxiety. There are several reasons for this:

- The compulsion draws the person's attention to the obsessive thought, making it more likely to recur.

- Compulsions are a form of safety behaviour. As we've seen, safety behaviours prevent us from discovering that our anxiety is exaggerated: someone who avoids physical contact with other people because they're afraid of contamination is unable to learn that you can't contract an illness by shaking hands.

- Compulsions frequently involve unrealistic targets. Regardless of the precautions we take, we can never be certain that an accident won't occur. No matter how long we spend washing and cleaning, absolute spotlessness is sure to elude us. The desire for cast-iron certainty leaves the person with OCD feeling that they could always do more – thereby fuelling their anxiety.

- Many compulsions are inherently counterproductive. For example, people with OCD often try to suppress their obsessions. But trying not to think about something can make it *more* likely that you'll do so, not less. (You can give this a go: try not to think about white bears.) And there's evidence that people with OCD are less able to suppress thoughts than other people.

- Repeated checking is a common feature of OCD. Yet checking doesn't bring certainty: in fact, the more a person (even someone without psychological problems) checks something, the less sure they become. This is because repeated checking reduces the vividness of our memory, though not its accuracy. And because the memory seems less vivid, we distrust it – and thus check again.

The cognitive behavioural therapy developed by Salkovskis and colleagues teaches the person with OCD to change the way they interpret their impulsive thoughts – to regard them as normal and inconsequential, rather than doom-laden reminders of personal responsibility – and to abandon the compulsions that fuel their anxiety.

Biological perspectives

Neurologically, OCD is distinct from the other anxiety disorders. The latter, as we saw in Chapter 2, are thought to involve problems in the amygdala, frontal lobes, and/or hippocampus. OCD, on the other hand, seems to be characterized by malfunction in a circuit comprising the orbitofrontal cortex, anterior cingulate cortex, striatum, and thalamus.

(Hoarding, incidentally, is thought to engage different areas of the brain – which is one of the reasons some scientists feel it shouldn't be categorized as a form of OCD. In fact, research led by David Mataix-Cols suggests that washing, checking, and hoarding each involve 'distinct but partially overlapping neural systems'.)

In especially severe cases of OCD – cases that respond neither to psychotherapy nor medication – surgery may be performed. (OCD is the only anxiety disorder to be treated by means of neurosurgery.) The operation, termed a cingulotomy, aims to break the OCD neurocircuit at the anterior cingulate. The success rate is moderate: a study of 44 patients operated on at Massachusetts General Hospital since 1989 found that 32% improved significantly, with a further 14% experiencing partial benefit. Some of these patients had undergone more than one cingulotomy.

OCD seems to run in families, though not to any great degree. Having a first-degree relative with OCD elevates your own risk of developing the disorder from around 3% to 7%. Genetic heritability is thought to be modest. Twin studies of OCD are rare, but some have found no evidence of heritability. On the other hand, a twin study of OCD-like symptoms estimated heritability at 36%.

Environmental perspectives

With genes making a relatively limited contribution to OCD, the spotlight falls onto environmental factors.

OCD has been linked to traumatic events in childhood (especially sexual abuse); relatively low socio-economic status; and hostile or neglectful parenting. However, these are also experiences that make a person vulnerable to anxiety disorders in general, and indeed to depression, alcohol and drug issues, and a wide range of psychiatric problems. The search for environmental influences specific to OCD continues.

Chapter 10
Post-traumatic stress disorder

Among the thousands of people who volunteered their help in the hours following the terrorist attacks on the World Trade Center on 11 September 2001 were many doctors. What they experienced was so distressing that, when approached by researchers 18 months later, most preferred to keep their thoughts to themselves. A few, however, did agree to talk. Lynn de Lisi collected their accounts:

> One particular physician, a female psychiatrist...experienced survivor guilt, and [felt] that she needed to be doing more. At the time of the interview, she still felt somewhat removed from other people and irritable, and had upsetting reminders that lingered.
>
> Another physician said he drank twice as much alcohol after September 11 than before. He worked at a triage unit close to the World Trade Center site volunteering about 10 hours per day....He stated that his worst memory was seeing people jump out of the towers.
>
> One physician was a staff psychiatrist on an inpatient unit who worked longer hours after the attacks. His alcohol intake increased after the attacks and at the time of the interview he still admitted to being preoccupied with painful images intruding on his thoughts. He still avoided participating in activities that would remind him of the events.

But it wasn't necessary to be directly involved for psychological problems to develop. Many Americans, even those living far from New York City, were profoundly shaken. Two months after 11 September, 17% of the 1,300 people contacted across the US in one survey reported associated post-traumatic stress symptoms. (Scale up that representative sample and you arrive at a total of 45 million people suffering serious psychological distress as a result of the attacks.) With the passing of time, the number of people reporting symptoms declined. Three years later, when 1,950 individuals were contacted by the same researchers, 4.5% were affected.

Overall, the people most likely to develop problems were those who had:

- personally witnessed the attacks;
- watched live television coverage;
- experienced traumatic events in their childhood, or after 11 September;
- suffered previously from a psychological disorder.

What is post-traumatic stress disorder?

Given the magnitude of the horror inflicted upon New Yorkers on 11 September, it's hardly surprising that many people – and especially those directly affected by the atrocity – subsequently developed severe psychological problems. But post-traumatic stress disorder (PTSD) is usually triggered by more commonplace disasters. The American Psychiatric Association's *Diagnostic and Statistical Manual* (*DSM*) defines a traumatic event as one in which:

the person experienced, witnessed, or was confronted with an event or events that involved actual or threatened death or serious injury, or a threat to the physical integrity of self or others.

Examples of such trauma include serious traffic accidents, sexual assault, physical attack, violent robbery or mugging, the sudden death of a loved one, military combat, torture, natural disasters, and being diagnosed with a potentially fatal illness.

PTSD is marked by three types of symptoms (that must persist for more than a month):

- *Reliving the traumatic event.* This can take the form of nightmares or flashbacks, when the person feels that they are right back in the midst of the horror. Thoughts of the trauma constantly recur, no matter how doggedly the person tries to forget. Distressing memories can be sparked by the smallest things – perhaps a particular sound or smell, a place, or the look on someone's face.

- *Avoiding any reminder of the traumatic event/feeling numb.* The memory of the trauma is so upsetting that sufferers will go to any lengths to avoid triggering it. They try to suppress thoughts of the event; they steer clear of people and places that could remind them of what happened; and they don't want to talk about their experiences. People with PTSD often report that they are emotionally 'numb' – at least to positive emotions like happiness. And they may try to deaden the anxiety and depression they feel by using alcohol or drugs. (Some experts argue that numbness is sufficiently different from avoidance to be regarded as a symptom category in its own right.)

- *Feeling constantly on edge.* This is what psychologists call a state of *hyperarousal*, and it means being always anxious, irritable, and tense. People with PTSD are constantly on the alert for any reminder of the trauma: it dominates their world, day and night (sleep problems are a typical symptom of PTSD).

Anxiety

As with all psychiatric diagnoses, however, many people may develop symptoms that aren't sufficiently severe, persistent, or numerous to meet the official criteria, but which cause much distress nonetheless. And some researchers have questioned the *DSM*'s interpretation of what constitutes a trauma, suggesting that negative life events such as chronic illness, divorce, or unemployment can generate at least as many symptoms of PTSD as rape, assault, accidents, and so on.

How common is PTSD?

A reliable picture of the prevalence of PTSD is provided by the US National Comorbidity Survey (NCS), which found that roughly 50% of people experience at least one trauma in their lifetime, with 7.8% of the total sample developing PTSD. The figure is not dramatically different for young people. Of the 10,000 13- to 18-year-olds interviewed for the US National Comorbidity Survey Replication Adolescent Supplement, 5% reported having experienced PTSD, with 1.5% severely affected.

Many types of trauma can trigger PTSD, but some are more potent than others. According to the NCS, the traumas most likely to result in PTSD in women were rape, sexual molestation, physical attack, being threatened with a weapon, and childhood physical abuse; and in men, rape, combat exposure, childhood neglect, and childhood physical abuse.

Women in the NCS were twice as likely to develop PTSD as men, even though they experienced fewer traumas. This is only partly explained by the fact that women are more likely to experience the kinds of trauma that commonly produce PTSD (rape, for example). Exposed to the same type of trauma, women are more likely than men to develop PTSD – for reasons that are currently unknown.

Research on PTSD in the developing world is scarce. But a team led by Joop de Jong investigated rates of the problem in four of the world's poorest, most conflict-ridden countries: Algeria, where appalling violence erupted after elections were cancelled in 1991; Cambodia, which endured civil war in the 1960s and then the murderous regime of the Khmer Rouge; Ethiopia, also wracked by civil war; and Gaza, site of recurrent conflict since Israeli occupation in 1967. One would expect rates of PTSD in these troubled countries to be higher than in the West, and so it proved: 37.4% in Algeria (where violence was still occurring at the time of de Jong's research); 28.4% in Cambodia; 15.8% in Ethiopia; and 17.8% in Gaza.

No one received a diagnosis of PTSD until 1980, when it was included in the *DSM* for the first time. The psychological effects of combat had been acknowledged since the First World War, when huge numbers of soldiers developed 'shell-shock'. But it took until the 1970s for PTSD to be recognized, largely through the efforts of Vietnam War veterans' organizations – the Vietnam War having generated many thousands of cases – and those working with rape survivors. In 1990, it was estimated that more than a million US veterans had developed PTSD as a result of their experiences in Vietnam, with 479,000 still battling the disorder.

What causes PTSD?

Psychological perspectives

In one sense, the cause of PTSD is obvious: a specific trauma. And yet this is only part of the explanation. Why is it that some people who are raped or badly beaten up develop PTSD and others do not?

Of the psychological attempts to answer that question, arguably the most influential is the one formulated by Anke Ehlers and David Clark.

The theory is nicely illustrated by a research study carried out by Ehlers and colleagues. For six months, they tracked the progress of 147 people who'd been injured in motor vehicle accidents. Two weeks after the accident, 33 (22.4%) met the criteria for a diagnosis of PTSD (except, of course, the stipulation that symptoms have lasted more than a month); six months later, 17 (12.1%) were affected.

The individuals who developed PTSD tended to share certain characteristics:

- *Before the accident*: a history of emotional problems and previous traumatic experiences.
- *During the accident*: a focus on the sensations evoked by the trauma, rather than the meaning of what was happening (this is called 'data-driven processing'); the feeling that the accident was happening to someone else (a lack of 'self-referential thinking'); a sensation of detachment or numbness or that the accident wasn't real.
- *After the accident*: a pessimistic view of the trauma; an inability to clearly recall what had gone on; a perceived lack of support from friends and family; constant thoughts of the accident and its consequences or, conversely, avoidance of all reminders; adoption of safety behaviours (for instance, refusing to travel by car).

Ehlers and Clark argue that PTSD arises when the person believes they are *still seriously threatened* in some way by the trauma they've experienced. Why should someone assume they are still endangered by an event that happened months or even years previously? Ehlers and Clark identify two factors.

First is a negative interpretation of the trauma and the normal feelings that follow, for example:

- Nowhere is safe.
- I attract disaster.

- I can't cope with stress.
- I'm going mad.
- I'll never be able to get over this.
- No one is there for me.

These interpretations can make the person feel in danger *physically* (the world seems fundamentally unsafe), or *psychologically* (their self-confidence and sense of wellbeing seem irreparably damaged).

Second are problems with the memory of the trauma. Because of the way the person reacts during the event, the memory somehow fails to acquire a properly developed context and meaning. As a result, it constantly intrudes, triggered automatically by the slightest reminder of the trauma (a colour, or smell, or vague physical resemblance). Ehlers and Clark liken the traumatic memory to:

> a cupboard in which many things have been thrown in quickly and in a disorganised fashion, so it is impossible to fully close the door and things fall out at unpredictable times.

(In a related theory, Chris Brewin argues that PTSD develops when unconscious, situationally accessible memories (SAMs) of the trauma – which largely comprise sensory information – fail to be incorporated in conscious, verbally accessible memory (VAMs).)

PTSD is maintained by exactly the kind of behaviours adopted by the individuals in the traffic accident study. Thus, cognitive therapy aims to persuade the person to drop these behaviours, and to tackle the negative beliefs and incomplete memories that provoke them.

Biological perspectives

PTSD seems to be marked by problems in the limbic system of the brain, and specifically the relationship between the:

- *amygdala*, the storehouse of unconscious fear memories;

- *anterior cingulate cortex* (ACC), which helps control our fear reactions;

- *hippocampus*, which stores contextual memories (for example, where we were and what we were doing when a frightening event occurred), and can therefore help us judge whether a situation is truly dangerous or merely resembles aspects of a previously threatening event.

In people suffering from PTSD, the amygdala may be overactive and the ACC and hippocampus underactive. Indeed, there's evidence to suggest that the ACC and hippocampus are actually smaller in people with PTSD, though whether that's a result of the illness or a cause is unclear. (In fact, it may not be the whole hippocampus that is affected; recent research has highlighted atrophy in a specific region of the hippocampus in people with PTSD.)

Without the moderating influence of the ACC and hippocampus, the amygdala may perceive threat where there is none – a hallmark of PTSD, and indeed of anxiety disorders in general.

It's been suggested that the hippocampus may shrink through the effects of the hormone cortisol. Cortisol, and related neurochemicals, are released via the hypothalamic-pituitary-adrenal (HPA) axis in order to key up the body to respond to potential threat. Scientists are investigating the idea that dysfunction in the HPA axis may play an important role in PTSD. So far, however, no consistent pattern has emerged.

Research into the genetics of PTSD is scarce. What there is suggests only moderate heritability (around the 30–35% mark). Interestingly, there seems to be some overlap between genetic susceptibility to PTSD and to some types of the trauma that trigger the illness. This may be a result of the individual's personality. Murray Stein and colleagues have speculated:

> an individual's genetically influenced propensity toward neuroticism would lead the individual to experience more anger and irritability, making that person 1) more likely to get into fights (thereby increasing the risk of experiencing assaultive trauma) and 2) more likely to become highly emotionally aroused as a result of experiencing such traumata (thereby increasing the risk for PTSD symptoms).

In some cases, then, personality may partly influence the likelihood of a person experiencing a trauma and of then developing PTSD. But we shouldn't get carried away: most traumatic events occur out of the blue and regardless of the individual's personality.

Chapter 11
Treatment

Around one-third of the adult population reports difficulties with anxiety, with close to one in five having problems severe enough to meet criteria for a clinical disorder. And anxiety can feel horrible, as Holly Golightly pointed out back in Chapter 1. Anxiety, then, can be a big problem. How are we faring for solutions?

In fact, simply establishing which treatments are effective is an immensely complex, labour-intensive business. The undoubted 'gold standard' for clinical research is what's known as randomized controlled trials. These involve participants being randomly assigned to one of at least two groups. Group one will receive a specific treatment, and group two either a 'control' non-treatment (a placebo, for example) or an alternative treatment. (Sometimes trials will assess two or more treatments against a control.) Allocating participants randomly means that the composition of each group should be similar, and by following their outcomes, you can see whether the treatment has helped, over and above natural recovery.

But even randomized controlled trials are not as straightforward as they can appear. This is why medical researchers are encouraged to follow the CONSORT (Consolidated Standards of Reporting Trials) guidelines. The latest CONSORT statement was issued in 2010, after seven years of consultations, and it has the backing of the leading medical journals (which is where most scientists hope to publish their results).

Among the numerous factors CONSORT urges researchers to consider when designing and reporting a trial are: the nature of the patients selected (for example, how severe their problem; how long-lasting it is; whether they have other problems); the techniques used to randomly allocate participants to treatment groups (there are several alternatives); the nature of the control treatment; the composition and quality of the treatment being tested; what types of outcome are measured; whether the research assessors and patients were blind to treatment allocation; what to do about people who drop out of the trial; length of follow-up after the treatment has concluded; appropriate statistical analysis – and so on. And on.

Unfortunately, not all clinical trials adhere to the CONSORT guidelines – and they didn't exist at all until 1996. And even the best trials can only tell us about particular durations or dosages of treatment for a particular group over a particular time period. This means that there are uncertainties and gaps in knowledge. Hence clinicians often debate the question: what works for whom?

What works?

Establishing the efficacy of specific treatments, then, is an inordinately tricky business. And yet in the case of anxiety disorders, we do have a consensus.

The number one treatment of choice is psychological therapy – principally cognitive behaviour therapy (CBT) and its variants. (We've highlighted the theoretical foundations of CBT in the chapters on specific disorders.) Anxiety occurs when we believe a situation is threatening. CBT's core objective is to test the accuracy of those beliefs. This is achieved by carefully exposing individuals to the situations and feelings that they fear in a way that allows them to learn from the experience. When the tests are carried out in a controlled, graduated, and individually tailored fashion, the person discovers that they are actually much safer than they had thought and their anxiety decreases.

But anxiety is also tackled with medication. For long-term treatment, SSRI antidepressants (such as paroxetine) are preferred. But in the short term, specific anxiolytic (anti-anxiety) drugs may be prescribed to help a patient cope with a crisis. The most commonly used anxiolytics are the benzodiazepines: these tend to work very rapidly and effectively, but can lead to tolerance (your body becomes used to the effects of the drug and therefore increasing doses are required) and to addiction – hence the recommendation that they only be used in the short term.

The gains brought about by CBT are sometimes greater, and typically last longer, than those produced by medication. Moreover, medication can sometimes produce side effects – and giving them up can be tricky. This is why the UK's National Institute for Clinical Excellence recommends CBT as the first line of treatment for each of the anxiety disorders, with SSRIs as a second choice. (We'll look at the various treatment alternatives in greater detail below.)

Interestingly, combining psychological therapy and medication doesn't seem to bring any additional benefits. In fact, in some cases (panic disorder, for instance), medication may actually interfere with the therapy. This is because, in order to learn that you can cope with your anxiety in a controlled exposure, it's necessary to really *feel* your fear – which is something anti-anxiety medication is intended, of course, to prevent.

One interesting development, however, is the use of drugs to boost the effects of psychological therapy. It is early days, but promising results have been obtained with 'cognitive enhancers' such as D-cycloserine (drugs that quicken learning). D-cycloserine appears to speed up the progress made when individuals test out the accuracy of their fearful thoughts.

What treatments are people receiving?

As we've seen, official guidelines in the UK advocate the use of CBT to treat anxiety disorders. But how many people with anxiety disorders are actually receiving CBT – or indeed any other form of treatment?

Not nearly enough, would seem to be the inevitable conclusion when you look at the data from a survey carried out for the NHS in 2007. Here are the percentages of people receiving no treatment at all:

- Generalized anxiety disorder: 66%
- Phobias: 43%
- Obsessive-compulsive disorder: 69%
- Panic disorder: 75%
- Mixed anxiety and depressive episode: 85%

Here are the figures for people with anxiety disorders receiving medication only:

- Generalized anxiety disorder: 18%
- Phobias: 23%
- Obsessive-compulsive disorder: 12%
- Panic disorder: 8%
- Mixed anxiety and depressive episode: 11%

And now the figures for people with anxiety disorders receiving some form of counselling or therapy, either with medication or on its own, with the figure in bold denoting CBT:

- Generalized anxiety disorder: 15%; **3%**
- Phobias: 34%; **11%**

- Obsessive-compulsive disorder: 18%; **4%**
- Panic disorder: 17%; **4%**
- Mixed anxiety and depressive episode: 5%; **1%**

One of the reasons CBT is so rarely used is a shortage of trained therapists. This is a situation the UK government has attempted to rectify by means of the Improving Access to Psychological Therapies scheme, which was launched in 2007 with the aim of training 3,600 new therapists.

Medication

Three main types of drugs are used to treat anxiety: SSRIs, benzodiazepines, and beta-blockers.

SSRIs

You might be surprised to discover that anxiety is treated with SSRIs (selective serotonin reuptake inhibitors). SSRIs, after all, are popularly regarded as anti-depressants. They were certainly marketed as anti-depressants when they appeared on the scene in the late 1980s. But their ability to dampen down feelings of anxiety has made them the primary pharmaceutical option for these disorders. Indeed, some experts have argued that they are more effective at treating anxiety than depression.

Among the SSRIs commonly prescribed for anxiety problems are paroxetine, venlafaxine, and sertraline. Unlike the other drug options, they often take a few weeks to show benefits. Once SSRIs kick in, however, they can reduce our sense of threat and instead stimulate a feeling of calm contentment. How they do this is unknown. SSRIs increase the amount of serotonin in the brain, but what this means for anxiety isn't well understood. As the psychiatrist David Healy has written: 'We know a lot about where drugs go in the brain but very little about how they work.'

Benzodiazepines

Like many other drugs, the success of benzodiazepines owed much to luck. A scientist named Leo Sternbach synthesized chlordiazepoxide in 1955 while working for the pharmaceutical giant Hoffmann-La Roche, but could see no reason to continue working on it.

Chlordiazepoxide sat in a corner of Sternbach's lab for two years until a colleague, Earl Reeder, took another look. Reeder was astonished by the results, and the company was quick to see the potential. Chlordiazepoxide, renamed Librium, was introduced to the market in 1960, followed a few years later by diazepam (Valium).

Benzodiazepines appeared to offer a safe, quick-acting cure for the effects of anxiety, and they were astonishingly popular. It's perhaps not surprising that the public were so keen: benzodiazepines produce a sense of relaxation that resembles the feeling produced by alcohol. They do this by enhancing the effect of a neurochemical called gamma aminobutyric acid (GABA), which relaxes us when we're anxious.

Gradually, however, it was recognized that all was not quite as rosy in the benzodiazepine garden as it seemed. Unpleasant side effects were common, and stopping the drug could result in nasty withdrawal symptoms. In fact, the tide of scientific and popular opinion turned so conclusively that the brand name Valium was dropped.

Benzodiazepines (also known as 'minor tranquillizers') are still widely prescribed for some anxiety problems, though are only recommended for short-term use: usually two to four weeks. Commonly used varieties include chlordiazepoxide (Librium) and diazepam (the former Valium), lorazepam

(Ativan), bromazepam (Lexotan), alprazolam (Xanax), and clorazepate (Tranxene).

Beta-blockers

At the 2008 Beijing Olympics, North Korean competitor Kim Jong-su became the first ever pistol shooter to be expelled from the Games after testing positive for a banned substance. The substance in question was the drug propanolol, a beta-blocker, and it cost Kim Jong-su his silver and bronze medals.

Why a pistol shooter might be tempted to take a beta-blocker is no mystery. These drugs – of which propanolol was the first to be developed, in the late 1950s – quickly prevent many of the physiological symptoms of anxiety, such as elevated heart rate, perspiration, and trembling.

Beta-blockers are principally prescribed to treat cardiovascular problems such as high blood pressure or angina. But they are thought to be widely used by orchestral musicians and other performers to control the effects of nerves. While beta-blockers may help with specific, short-term situations, they aren't recommended for long-term treatment of anxiety disorders.

Cognitive behaviour therapy

CBT was developed by the American psychiatrist Aaron Beck (born 1921), initially as a treatment for depression. As the psychologist Gillian Butler has written, CBT is 'based on the recognition that thoughts and feelings are closely related. If you *think* something is going to go wrong, you will *feel* anxious; if you *think* everything will go fine, you will *feel* more confident.' So CBT therapists work with their clients to identify and evaluate negative thoughts and the unhelpful behaviours that often result.

CBT isn't a narrowly prescriptive programme. Exactly how it is applied to anxiety (or indeed any other problem) depends on the nature of the disorder and the person being treated. Treatment is based on the construction of detailed models showing how a disorder is caused, maintained, and overcome. As more is discovered, the model is updated and the therapy evolves accordingly.

(Incidentally, one of the problems commonly treated with CBT is *hypochondriasis*, which is the fear that one is suffering from a serious illness. Hypochondriasis is often referred to as 'health anxiety'. The psychiatric classification systems, however, don't categorize it as an anxiety disorder, though many experts believe it would be more logical to do so.)

At the core of CBT for anxiety is the idea that fear is a product of *interpretation*. We are frightened not because something awful is happening, but because we *believe* it will happen in the future. To overcome your anxiety, you must test out your interpretation by experiencing the situation you fear. And you must do so without adopting any of the safety behaviours you would ordinarily use in order to cope. If you can do that, you will discover that your fears are misplaced.

For example, a person suffering from OCD who fears contamination would be encouraged to seek out dirty environments, and to resist the compulsion to wash repeatedly afterwards as they would ordinarily do. An individual with panic disorder might be asked to visit a place they would usually avoid and to stay there even when they feel the sensations of panic. If they can ride out the panic, rather than fighting it, they'll find out that what they dreaded – a heart attack, perhaps, or fainting – didn't occur. And a person with social phobia might be shown videos of themselves in a social situation, once when using their safety behaviours (avoiding eye contact, for example, or carefully rehearsing everything they say) and once without those safety behaviours. They can then see that their safety behaviours aren't in fact helping. They'll probably also discover that they come across much better than they had imagined. Below we describe CBT for two problems in a little more depth.

CBT for phobias

CBT has been used very successfully to tackle a wide range of phobias. One notable example is the programme developed by Lars-Göran Öst, Professor of Psychology at the University of Stockholm, to treat people with a spider phobia. The programme is extremely brief, comprising just a one-hour assessment followed by a three-hour exposure session.

During those three hours, Öst guides the individual through a series of increasingly demanding tasks. As is normal in CBT exposure, Öst models the required behaviour for the client. Letting the person see exactly what's involved before they attempt a task helps encourage and relax them.

First, the person is taught to catch a small spider in a glass bowl; then to touch the spider; and finally to let the spider walk on their hand. Before the second task, the person is asked what they expect will happen. Öst notes: 'Almost 100 per cent of our patients say that the spider will crawl up on their hands, up the arm and underneath the clothes.' But the individual soon discovers that their interpretation is mistaken: in fact, the spider runs away.

Once the client has completed the three tasks, they repeat them with a series of increasingly large spiders. By the end of the session, the person will have the two biggest spiders walking around on their hands – a pretty remarkable achievement considering how they felt about spiders just a few hours previously.

Öst has developed a similar treatment for people suffering from blood-injection-injury phobias. In this case, clients are shown a series of increasingly gory images of wounds, operations, and the like. But these phobias are unlike any others: rather than the individual's blood pressure rising when confronted by the feared object or situation, it drops. And so, to prevent the person fainting when they see blood, Öst teaches them to detect the earliest signs of a fall in blood pressure and to respond by repeatedly tensing their muscles. This 'applied tension' increases the individual's blood pressure, thus enabling them to proceed with the exposure task.

CBT for post-traumatic stress disorder

State-of-the-art CBT for post-traumatic stress disorder (PTSD) typically has three objectives:

- To help the person to stop reliving the trauma by addressing their incomplete and chaotic memory of the event.
- To change the negative views the person holds about the trauma and what it means for them.
- To help the person to no longer avoid reminders of the trauma, or to numb their feelings with alcohol or drugs.

Treatment normally involves ten to twelve weekly ninety-minute sessions, followed by three monthly 'booster' sessions. This requires a very significant commitment of time (and emotion) on the part of the client. But a team of renowned CBT developers – Nick Grey, Freda McManus, Ann Hackmann, David Clark, and Anke Ehlers – has piloted an intensive course of treatment for PTSD, with sessions concentrated into one week. Let's look at an example from them.

Mark, a 31-year-old professional, had been suffering from nightmares, flashbacks, anger, and depression following a motorbike accident nine months previously. He felt so distressed and low that he contemplated suicide every day.

During the first part of the week, Mark was encouraged to 'relive' the accident in his imagination. His most upsetting memories were of sliding down the road after being hit by a car; the looming bus which he had believed would run him over; and lying in the road after the accident. Accompanying these memories were some very negative thoughts. He believed, for example, that his life was 'full of crap', and that the image of him lying alone on the ground epitomized his general isolation.

As the sessions progressed, Mark was helped both to fill in the gaps in his memory of the trauma and to challenge his negative thoughts. He remembered, for example, that several passers-by had been helpful and attentive, and that he'd lain alone in the road for much less time than he'd previously believed. Through discussions with the therapist, Mark came to see that his life was far from as bleak as he sometimes felt it was, and that he wasn't alone.

Mark was also encouraged to revisit the site of the accident – something he had always avoided. He began to ride his motorbike again. And for the first time, he was able to discuss his experience with his girlfriend.

A week after therapy, Mark's symptoms were greatly improved. And the gains lasted: 18 months later, Mark was still well and enjoying life.

Virtual-reality CBT

The exposure element within CBT works, but it's not without its drawbacks. It's suspected, for example, that some people are so reluctant to experience the situation they fear that they don't seek treatment. And how does one easily create exposure situations for someone who is afraid of flying?

One solution is virtual-reality (VR) CBT. This involves the individual wearing a specially designed headset that immerses them in a computer-generated representation of whatever it is they fear, complete with sounds, and sometimes even smells. VR has been used to treat panic disorder, social phobia, and fears of flying, spiders, and heights with similar success to normal '*in vivo*' exposure therapy. VR CBT is now being tested as a possible therapy for US veterans suffering from PTSD following service in Iraq and Afghanistan.

Self-help CBT

As a look around any decent-sized bookshop will tell you, self-help is big business. But does 'self-help' – and specifically CBT-based material – *really* help?

Before we answer that question, it's worth pointing out that these days self-help comes in several varieties. There are the traditional books – offering what's known as *bibliotherapy*; CD-ROMs; audio tapes; and Internet-based resources.

There's certainly no disputing the demand: many self-help books have gone on to become bestsellers, and the US National Institute of Mental Health reports seven million hits on its website every month. For many people, self-help is a much more palatable method of tackling their psychological problems than seeking advice from a health professional. And those same health professionals often recommend that their patients consult self-help materials as part of their treatment.

Which brings us back to that key question: does CBT-based self-help work? The evidence suggests that it can do, at least to some extent. But it tends to be much more effective when there's also input from a therapist in person.

Lifestyle

If you're concerned about your anxiety levels, a few changes to your lifestyle may well improve your mood a lot over time.

Well-controlled studies in this area are not plentiful, but there is evidence to suggest that anxiety can be lessened by:

- aerobic exercise;
- healthy diet;
- relaxation training (in which you learn to progressively relax your muscles);
- massage;
- yoga;
- mindfulness (a synthesis of modern Western psychological thinking and ancient Buddhist beliefs and practices, particularly meditation, that emphasizes learning to live in the moment, and understanding that your thoughts and feelings are temporary, transient, and not necessarily a reflection of reality).

A telling illustration of the difference the first two on this list can make was provided by a two-year study of more than 10,000 people living in some of the poorest areas of Britain. Large increases in the amount of physical exercise taken *or* the quantity of fruit and vegetables eaten led to significant improvements in mental health. In particular, people reported feeling much more peaceful and happy.

Anxiety can cause major difficulties for many people. But, as we've seen, there are now many ways of dealing with problematic anxiety. Some have been recognized for centuries; some were discovered by chance; and some of the most promising are based on the research into the causes of anxiety we've described in this book.

Appendix

Self-assessment questionnaires and further information

This Appendix contains self-assessment questionnaires for:

- social phobia
- generalized anxiety disorder (GAD)
- obsessive-compulsive disorder (OCD)
- post-traumatic stress disorder (PTSD)

It's important to bear in mind that these questionnaires won't provide a cast-iron diagnosis – for that, you'd need to see a specialist. However, they will give you an indication as to whether it may be useful to seek professional advice. For more information on treatment options, see Chapter 11.

In the Further reading section, you'll find a list of books and websites providing more information on each of the six main psychological disorders.

Social phobia

When you complete the following questionnaire, base your answers on your experiences over the past week.

A total score of 19 or more is a sign of possible social phobia.

0 = Not at all   1 = A little bit

2 = Somewhat   3 = Very much

4 = Extremely

1.	I am afraid of people in authority.	0	1	2	3	4
2.	I am bothered by blushing in front of people.	0	1	2	3	4
3.	Parties and social events scare me.	0	1	2	3	4
4.	I avoid talking to people I don't know.	0	1	2	3	4
5.	Being criticized scares me a lot.	0	1	2	3	4
6.	Fear of embarrassment causes me to avoid doing things or speaking to people.	0	1	2	3	4
7.	Sweating in front of people causes me distress.	0	1	2	3	4
8.	I avoid going to parties.	0	1	2	3	4
9.	I avoid activities in which I am the centre of attention.	0	1	2	3	4
10.	Talking to strangers scares me.	0	1	2	3	4
11.	I avoid having to give speeches.	0	1	2	3	4
12.	I would do anything to avoid being criticized.	0	1	2	3	4
13.	Heart palpitations bother me when I am around people.	0	1	2	3	4
14.	I am afraid of doing things when people might be watching.	0	1	2	3	4
15.	Being embarrassed or looking stupid are my worst fears.	0	1	2	3	4
16.	I avoid speaking to anyone in authority.	0	1	2	3	4
17.	Trembling or shaking in front of others is distressing to me.	0	1	2	3	4

Social Phobia Inventory © 2000 Royal College of Psychiatrists

Generalized anxiety disorder

If you're concerned that your worrying might be getting out of control, try the Penn State Worry Questionnaire.

For each of the following statements, indicate how typical or characteristic they are for you by giving a score from 1 to 5.

1	2	3	4	5
Not at all typical		Somewhat typical		Very typical

1. If I don't have enough time to do everything, I don't worry about it.   1 2 3 4 5

2. My worries overwhelm me.   1 2 3 4 5

3. I don't tend to worry about things.   1 2 3 4 5

4. Many situations make me worry.   1 2 3 4 5

5. I know I shouldn't worry about things, but I just can't help it.   1 2 3 4 5

6. When I'm under pressure, I worry a lot.   1 2 3 4 5

7. I am always worrying about something.   1 2 3 4 5

8. I find it easy to dismiss worrisome thoughts.   1 2 3 4 5

9. As soon as I finish one task, I start to worry about something else.   1 2 3 4 5

10. I never worry about anything.   1 2 3 4 5

11. When there is nothing more I can do about a concern, I don't worry about it any more.   1 2 3 4 5

12. I've been a worrier all my life.   1 2 3 4 5

13. I notice that I have been worrying about things.   1 2 3 4 5

14. Once I start worrying, I can't stop.   1 2 3 4 5

15. I worry all the time.   1 2 3 4 5

16. I worry about projects until they are all done.   1 2 3 4 5

Penn State Worry Questionnaire: Meyer, T. J., Miller, M. L., Metzger, R. L., and Borkovec, T. D., (1990). Development and validation of the Penn State Worry Questionnaire, *Behaviour Research and Therapy*, 28: 487–95.

Now add up your scores for each statement. Questions 3, 8, 10, and 11 are *reversed scored*: if, for example, you put 5, for scoring purposes the item is counted as 1. Scores can range from 18 to 80.

People with worry problems usually score above 50. A score of over 60 may indicate GAD.

Obsessive-compulsive disorder

When you answer the following questions, think back to your experiences over the past month.

0 = Not at all   1 = A little
2 = Moderately   3 = A lot
4 = Extremely

1. I have saved up so many things that they get in the way.   0   1   2   3   4
2. I check things more often than necessary.   0   1   2   3   4
3. I get upset if objects are not arranged properly.   0   1   2   3   4
4. I feel compelled to count while I am doing things.   0   1   2   3   4
5. I find it difficult to touch an object when I know it has been touched by strangers or certain people.   0   1   2   3   4
6. I find it difficult to control my own thoughts.   0   1   2   3   4
7. I collect things I don't need.   0   1   2   3   4
8. I repeatedly check doors, windows, drawers, etc.   0   1   2   3   4
9. I get upset if others change the way I have arranged things.   0   1   2   3   4
10. I feel I have to repeat certain numbers.   0   1   2   3   4
11. I sometimes have to wash or clean myself simply because I feel contaminated.   0   1   2   3   4
12. I am upset by unpleasant thoughts that come into my mind against my will.   0   1   2   3   4

13.	I avoid throwing things away because I am afraid I might need them later.	0 1 2 3 4
14.	I repeatedly check gas and water taps and light switches after turning them off.	0 1 2 3 4
15.	I need things to be arranged in a particular order.	0 1 2 3 4
16.	I feel that there are good and bad numbers.	0 1 2 3 4
17.	I wash my hands more often and longer than necessary.	0 1 2 3 4
18.	I frequently get nasty thoughts and have difficulty in getting rid of them.	0 1 2 3 4

Questionnaire reproduced by permission of Edna B. Foa 2002.

Add up your score. A total of 21 or above indicates possible OCD.

Post-traumatic stress disorder

For this questionnaire, please base your responses on your reaction over the past seven days to the traumatic event.

As we saw in Chapter 10, there are three main types of PTSD symptom:

- *Reliving the traumatic event* is measured by items 1, 2, 3, 6, 9, 14, 16, 20. Scores can range from 0 to 32.
- *Avoidance or feeling numb* is measured by items 5, 7, 8, 11, 12, 13, 17, 22. Again, scores can range from 0 to 32.
- *Feeling constantly on edge* is measured by items 4, 10, 15, 18, 19, 21. Scores can range from 0 to 24.

The higher the scores, the more likely it is that you may be suffering from PTSD. Some experts estimate a total score of 30 or higher for the whole questionnaire indicates possible PTSD, but, as with all the questionnaires in this Appendix, a diagnosis can only be made by a clinician after a detailed assessment.

0 = Not at all   1 = A little bit
2 = Moderately   3 = Quite a bit
4 = Extremely

1. Any reminder brought back feelings about it.	0	1	2	3	4
2. I had trouble staying asleep.	0	1	2	3	4
3. Other things kept making me think about it.	0	1	2	3	4
4. I felt irritable and angry.	0	1	2	3	4
5. I avoided letting myself get upset when I thought about it or was reminded of it.	0	1	2	3	4
6. I thought about it when I didn't mean to.	0	1	2	3	4
7. I felt as if it hadn't happened or wasn't real.	0	1	2	3	4
8. I stayed away from reminders about it.	0	1	2	3	4
9. Pictures about it popped into my mind.	0	1	2	3	4
10. I was jumpy and easily startled.	0	1	2	3	4
11. I tried not to think about it.	0	1	2	3	4
12. I was aware that I still had a lot of feelings about it, but I didn't deal with them.	0	1	2	3	4
13. My feelings about it were kind of numb.	0	1	2	3	4
14. I found myself acting or feeling like I was back at that time.	0	1	2	3	4
15. I had trouble falling asleep.	0	1	2	3	4
16. I had waves of strong feelings about it.	0	1	2	3	4
17. I tried to remove it from my memory.	0	1	2	3	4
18. I had trouble concentrating.	0	1	2	3	4
19. Reminders of it caused me to have physical reactions, such as sweating, trouble breathing, nausea, or a pounding heart.	0	1	2	3	4
20. I had dreams about it.	0	1	2	3	4
21. I felt watchful and on guard.	0	1	2	3	4
22. I tried not to talk about it.	0	1	2	3	4

Impact of Event Scale – Revised © Weiss, D. S., and Marmar, C. R. (1997).

Appendix

Appendix acknowledgements

Social phobia questionnaire reproduced from Connor, K., Davidson, J., Churchill L., Sherwood, A., Weisler, R., & Foa, E., 'Psychometric properties of the Social Phobia Inventory'. *British Journal of Psychiatry* (2000), 176, 379–386 with permission from The Royal College of Psychiatrists © 2000 The Royal College of Psychiatrists.

Generalized anxiety disorder questionnaire reproduced from Meyer, T.J., Metzger, R.L. & Borkovec, T.D., 'Development and validation of the Penn State Worry Questionnaire'. *Behaviour Research and Therapy* (1990), 28, 487–495 with permission from © Elsevier.

Obsessive-compulsive disorder questionnaire reproduced with permission from Professor Edna B. Foa (2002).

Post-traumatic stress disorder questionnaire reproduced from Weiss, D.S. & Marmar, C.R., 'The Impact of Event Scale – Revised' in Wilson, J. & Keane, T.M. (eds) *Assessing Psychological Trauma and PTSD* (1997) pp. 399–411, New York: Guilford with permission from Professors Daniel S. Weiss and Charles Marmar.

Anxiety

Sources

Chapter 1

American Psychiatric Association. (2000). *Diagnostic and Statistical Manual of Mental Disorders*, 4th edn., Text Revision. (Arlington, VA: American Psychiatric Association).

Arrindell, W.A., Emmelkamp, P.M.G. and Van der Ende, J. (1984). Phobic Dimensions—I. Reliability and Generalizability across Samples, Gender and Nations. *Advances in Behaviour Research and Therapy*, 6: 207–254.

Banse, R. and Scherer, K.R. (1996). Acoustic Profiles in Vocal Emotion Expression. *Journal of Personality and Social Psychology*, 70: 614–636.

Barlow, D.H. (2002). *Anxiety and its Disorders*, 2nd edn. (New York: Guilford Press).

Berrios, G. & Porter, R. (eds.) (1995). *A History of Clinical Psychiatry: The Origin and History of Psychiatric Disorders*. (London: Athlone Press).

Dalgleish, T. and Power, M. (1999). *Handbook of Cognition and Emotion*. (Chichester: Wiley).

Darwin, C. (1872/1999). *The Expression of the Emotions in Man and Animals*. (London: Fontana).

Edelmann, R.J. (1992). *Anxiety*. (Chichester: Wiley).

Ekman, P. (1992). An Argument for Basic Emotions. *Cognition and Emotion*, 6, 169–200.

Hertenstein, M., Keltner, D., App, B., Bulleit, B.A., and Jaskolka, A.R. (2006). Touch Communicates Distinct Emotions. *Emotion*, 6: 528–533.

Kessler, R.C., Chiu, W.T., Demler, O. and Walters, E.E. (2005). Prevalence, Severity, and Comorbidity of 12-Month *DSM-IV* Disorders in the National Comorbidity Survey Replication. *Archives of General Psychiatry*, 62: 617–627.

Lewis, A. (1970). The Ambiguous Word 'Anxiety'. *International Journal of Psychiatry*, 9: 62–79.

Oatley, K., Keltner, D., and Jenkins, J.M. (2006). *Understanding Emotions*, 2nd edn. (Oxford: Blackwell).

Power, M. and Dalgleish, T. (1997). *Cognition and Emotion: From Order to Disorder*. (Hove: Psychology Press).

Rachman, S. (2004). *Anxiety*, 2nd edn. (Hove and New York: Psychology Press).

Susskind, J.M., Lee, D.H., Cusi, A., Feiman, R., Grabski, W. and Anderson, A.K. (2008). Expressing Fear Enhances Sensory Acquisition. *Nature Neuroscience*, 11: 843–850.

Tuma, A.H. and Maser, J.D. (eds) (1985). *Anxiety and the Anxiety Disorders*. (New Jersey: Lawrence Erlbaum Associates).

Chapter 2

Barlow, D.H. (2002). *Anxiety and its Disorders*, 2nd edn. (New York: Guilford Press).

Barlow, D.H. and Durand, V.M. (2005). *Abnormal Psychology: An Integrative Approach*. (Belmont, CA: Thomson Wadsworth).

Beck, A.T. and Emery, G. (1985). *Anxiety Disorders and Phobias: A Cognitive Perspective*. (Cambridge, MA.: Basic Books).

Bishop, S.J. (2007). Neurocognitive Mechanisms of Anxiety: An Integrative Approach. *Trends in Cognitive Sciences*, 11: 307–316.

Britton, J.C. and Rauch, S.L. (2009). Neuroanatomy and Neuroimaging of Anxiety Disorders. In M.M. Antony and M.B. Stein (eds.), *Oxford Handbook of Anxiety and Related Disorders*. (New York: Oxford University Press).

Cannistraro, P.A. and Rauch, S.L. (2003). Neural Circuitry of Anxiety: Evidence from Structural and Functional Neuroimaging Studies. *Psychopharmacology Bulletin*, 37: 8–25.

Charney, D.C. and Nestler, E.J. (2004). *Neurobiology of Mental Illness*, 2nd edn. (New York: Oxford University Press).

Clark, D.A. and Beck, A.T. (2010). *Cognitive Therapy of Anxiety Disorders*. (New York: Guilford).

Clark, D.M. (1999). Anxiety Disorders: Why They Persist and How to Treat Them. *Behaviour Research and Therapy*, 37: S5-27.

Damasio, A.R., Grabowski, T.J., Bechara, A., Damasio, H., Ponto, L.L.B., Parvizi, J., and Hichwa, R.D. (2000). Subcortical and Cortical Brain Activity during the Feeling of Self-generated Emotions. *Nature Neuroscience*, 3: 1049–1056.

Edelmann, R.J. (1992). *Anxiety*. (Chichester: Wiley).

Freud S. (1895/1979). On the Grounds for Detaching a Particular Syndrome from Neurasthenia under the Description 'Anxiety Neurosis', in *On Psychopathology* (London: Penguin).

Freud, S. (1933/1991). Anxiety and Instinctual Life, in *New Introductory Lectures on Psychoanalysis*, vol. 2. (London: Penguin).

Gray, J.A. and McNaughton, N. (2000). *The Neuropsychology of Anxiety*, 2nd edn. (Oxford: Oxford University Press).

Holmes, E.A. and Mathews, A. (2005). Mental Imagery and Emotion: A Special Relationship? *Emotion*, 5: 489–497.

LeDoux, J. (1998). *The Emotional Brain*. (New York: Phoenix).

Mathews, A., Richards, A., and Eysenck, M. (1989). Interpretation of Homophones Related to Threat in Anxiety States. *Journal of Abnormal Psychology*, 98: 31–34.

Mowrer, O.H. (1939). A Stimulus-Response Analysis of Anxiety and Its Role as a Reinforcing Agent. *Psychological Review*, 46: 553–565.

Oatley, K., Keltner, D., and Jenkins, J.M. (2006). *Understanding Emotions*, 2nd edn. (Oxford: Blackwell).

Rachman, S. (2004). *Anxiety*, 2nd edn. (Hove and New York: Psychology Press).

Rose, S. (2011). Self Comes to Mind: Constructing the Conscious Brain by Antonio Damasio. *The Guardian*, 12 February 2011.

Salkovskis, P. (ed.) (1996). *The Frontiers of Cognitive Therapy*. (New York: Guilford).

Sheehy, N. (2004). *Fifty Key Thinkers in Psychology*. (London and New York: Routledge).

Watson, J. and Raynor, R. (1920). Conditioned Emotional Reactions. *Journal of Genetic Psychology*, 37: 394–419.

Chapter 3

Barlow, D.H. (2002). *Anxiety and its Disorders*, 2nd edn. (New York: Guilford Press).

Barlow, D.H. and Durand, V.M. (2005). *Abnormal Psychology: An Integrative Approach*. (Belmont, CA: Thomson Wadsworth).

Caspi, A. and Moffitt, T.E. (2006). Gene–Environment Interactions in Psychiatry: Joining Forces with Neuroscience. *Nature Reviews Neuroscience*, 7: 583–590.

Clark, D.A. and Beck, A.T. (2010). *Cognitive Therapy of Anxiety Disorders*. (New York: Guilford).

Eley, T.C., Gregory, A.M., Lau, J.Y.F., McGuffin, P., Napolitano, M., Rijsdijk, F., and Clark, D.M. (2008). In the Face of Uncertainty: A Twin Study of Ambiguous Information, Anxiety and Depression in Children. *Journal of Abnormal Child Psychology*, 36: 55–65.

Eley, T.C., Gregory, A.M., Clark, D.M., and Ehlers, A. (2007). Feeling Anxious: A Twin Study of Panic/Somatic Ratings, Anxiety Sensitivity and Heartbeat Perception in Children. *Journal of Child Psychology and Psychiatry* 48: 1184–1191.

Gerull, F.C. and Rappe, R.M. (2002). Mother Knows Best: Effects of Maternal Modeling on the Acquisition of Fear and Avoidance Behavior in Toddlers. *Behaviour Research and Therapy*, 40: 279–287.

Gelernter, J. and Stein, M.B. (2009). Heritability and Genetics of Anxiety Disorders. In M.M. Antony and M.B. Stein (eds.), *Oxford Handbook of Anxiety and Related Disorders*. (New York: Oxford University Press).

Hudson, J.L. and Rapee, R.M. (2009). Familial and Social Environments in the Etiology and Maintenance of Anxiety Disorders. In M.M. Antony and M.B. Stein (eds.), *Oxford Handbook of Anxiety and Related Disorders*. (New York: Oxford University Press).

Hettema, J.M., An, S.S., Neale, M.C., Bukszar, J., van den Oord, E.J., Kendler, K.S., and Chen, X. (2006). Association Between Glutamic Acid Decarboxylase Genes and Anxiety Disorders, Major Depression, and Neuroticism. *Molecular Psychiatry*, 11: 752–762.

Hettema, J.M., Neale, M.C., and Kendler, K.S. (2001). A Review and Metaanalysis of the Genetic Epidemiology of Anxiety Disorders. *American Journal of Psychiatry*, 158: 1568–1578.

LeDoux, J. (1998). *The Emotional Brain*. (New York: Phoenix).

Plaisier, I., de Bruijn, J.G.M., de Graaf, R., ten Have, M., Beekman, A.T.F., and Penninx, B.W.J.H. (2007). The Contribution of Working Conditions and Social Support to the Onset of Depressive and Anxiety Disorders among Male and Female Employees. *Social Science and Medicine*, 64: 401–410.

Plomin, R., DeFries, J.C., McClearn, G.E., and McGuffin, P. (2008). *Behavioral Genetics*, 5th edn. (New York: Worth).

Poulton, R., Andrews, G., and Millichamp, J. (2008). Gene-Environment Interaction and the Anxiety Disorders. *European Archives of Psychiatry and Clinical Neuroscience*, 258: 65–68.

Smoller, J.W., Gardner-Schuster, E., and Misiaszek, M. (2008). Genetics of Anxiety. *Depression and Anxiety*, 25: 368–377.

Stein, M.B., Schork, N.J., and Gelernter, J. (2008). Gene-by-Environment (Serotonin Transporter and Childhood Maltreatment) Interaction for Anxiety Sensitivity, an Intermediate Phenotype for Anxiety Disorders. *Neuropsychopharmacology*, 33: 312–319.

Stein, M.B., Walker, J.R., Anderson, G., Hazen, A.L., Ross, C.A., Eldridge, G., and Forde, D.R. (1996). Childhood Physical and Sexual Abuse in Patients with Anxiety Disorders in a Community Sample. *American Journal of Psychiatry*, 153: 275–277.

Warren, S.L., Huston, L., Egeland, B., and Sroufe, L.A. (1997). Child and Adolescent Anxiety Disorders and Early Attachment. *Journal of the American Academy of Child and Adolescent Psychiatry*, 36: 637–644.

Chapter 4

Smits, J.A.J., Berry, A.C., Rosenfield, D., Powers, M.B., Behar, E., and Otto, M.W. (2008). Reducing Anxiety Sensitivity with Exercise. *Depression and Anxiety*, 25: 689–699.

Spurr, J.M. and Stopa, L. (2002). Self-focused Attention in Social Phobia and Social Anxiety. *Clinical Psychology Review*, 22: 947–975.

Wilson, J. (2008). *Inverting the Pyramid: The History of Football Tactics* (London: Orion).

Chapter 5

American Psychiatric Association. (2000). *Diagnostic and Statistical Manual of Mental Disorders*, 4th edn., Text Revision. (Arlington, VA: American Psychiatric Association).

Barlow, D.H. (2002). *Anxiety and its Disorders*, 2nd edn. (New York: Guilford Press).

Cook, M. and Mineka, S. (1990). Selective Associations in the Observational Conditioning of Fear in Rhesus Monkeys. *Journal of Experimental Psychology: Animal Behavior Processes*, 16: 372–389.

Curtis, G.C., Magee, W.J., Eaton, W.W., Wittchen, H.-U., and Kessler, R.C. (1998). Specific Fears and Phobias: Epidemiology and Classification. *British Journal of Psychiatry*, 173: 212–217.

Davey, G. (2008). *Psychopathology: Research, Assessment, and Treatment in Clinical Psychology* (Chichester: Wiley-Blackwell).

Doogan, S. and Thomas, G.V. (1992). Origins of Fear of Dogs in Adults and Children: The Role of Conditioning Processes and Prior Familiarity with Dogs. *Behaviour Research and Therapy*, 30: 387–394.

Hettema, J.M., Annas, P., Neale, M.C., Kendler, K.S., and Fredrikson, M. (2003). A Twin Study of the Genetics of Fear Conditioning. *Archives of General Psychiatry*, 60: 702–708.

Jones, M.K. and Menzies, R.G. (2000). Danger Expectancies, Self-Efficacy, and Insight in Spider Phobia. *Behaviour Research and Therapy*, 38: 585–600.

Kendler, K.S., Myers, J., Prescott, C.A., and Neale, M.C. (2001). The Genetic Epidemiology of Irrational Fears and Phobias in Men. *Archives of General Psychiatry*, 58: 257–265.

Kessler, R.C., McGonagle, K.A., Zhao, S., Nelson, C.B., Hughes, M., Eshleman, S., Wittchen, H.-U., and Kendler, K.S. (1994). Lifetime and 12-Month Prevalence of *DSM-III-R* Psychiatric Disorders in the United States. *Archives of General Psychiatry*, 51: 8–19.

Kessler, R.C., Chiu, W.T., Demler, O., and Walters, E.E. (2005). Prevalence, Severity, and Comorbidity of 12-Month DSM-IV Disorders in the National Comorbidity Survey Replication. *Archives of General Psychiatry*, 62: 617–627.

LeDoux, J. (1998). Fear and the Brain: Where Have We Been and Where Are We Going? *Biological Psychiatry*, 44: 1229–1238.

McLean, C.P. and Anderson, E.R. (2009). Brave Men and Timid Women? A Review of the Gender Differences in Fear and Anxiety. *Clinical Psychology Review*, 29: 496–505.

McManus, S., Meltzer, H., Brugha, T., Bebbington, P., and Jenkins, R. (eds.) (2009) *Adult Psychiatric Morbidity in England, 2007: Results of a Household Survey*. (NHS Information Centre for Health and Social Care).

McNally, R.J. (1997). Atypical Phobias. In G.C.L. Davey (ed.), *Phobias: A Handbook of Theory, Research and Treatment* (Chichester: Wiley).

Öhman, A. and Mineka, S. (2001). Fears, Phobias, and Preparedness: Toward an Evolved Module of Fear and Fear Learning. *Psychological Review*, 108: 483–522.

Öst, L.-G. and Hugdahl, K. (1981). Acquisition of Phobias and Anxiety Response Patterns in Clinical Patients. *Behaviour Research and Therapy*, 19: 439–447.

Pierce, K.A. and Kirkpatrick, D.R. (1992). Do Men Lie on Fear Surveys? *Behaviour Research and Therapy*, 30: 415–418.

Plomin, R., DeFries, J.C., McClearn, G.E., and McGuffin, P. (2008). *Behavioral Genetics*, 5th edn. (New York: Worth).

Spitzer, R.L., Gibbon, M., Skodol, A.E., Williams, J.B.W., and First, M.B. (eds.) (2002). *DSM-IV-TR Casebook* (Washington and London: American Psychiatric Association).

Chapter 6

American Psychiatric Association. (2000). *Diagnostic and Statistical Manual of Mental Disorders*, 4th edn., Text Revision. (Arlington, VA: American Psychiatric Association).

Barlow, D.H. (2002). *Anxiety and its Disorders*, 2nd edn. (New York: Guilford Press).

Blair, K., Geraci, M., Devido, J., McCaffrey, D., Chen, G., Vythilingam, M., Ng, P., Hollon, N., Jones, M., Blair, R.J.R., and Pine, D.S. (2008). Neural Response to Self- and Other Referential Praise and Criticism in Generalized Social Phobia. *Archives of General Psychiatry*, 65: 1176–1184.

Clark, D.M. and Fairburn, C.G. (eds.) *Science and Practice of Cognitive Behaviour Therapy* (Oxford and New York: Oxford University Press).

Dannahy, L. and Stopa, L. (2007). Post-event Processing in Social Anxiety. *Behaviour Research and Therapy*, 45: 1207–1219.

Gilbert, P. (2000). The Relationship of Shame, Social Anxiety and Depression: The Role of the Evaluation of Social Rank. *Clinical Psychology and Psychotherapy*, 7: 174–189.

Hackmann, A., Surawy, C., and Clark, D.M. (1998). Seeing Yourself Through Others' Eyes: A Study of Spontaneously Occurring Images in Social Phobia. *Behavioural and Cognitive Psychotherapy*, 26: 3–12.

Hallett, V., Ronald, A., Rijsdijk, F., and Eley, T.C. (2009). Phenotypic and Genetic Differentiation of Anxiety-Related Behaviors in Middle Childhood. *Depression and Anxiety*, 26: 316–324.

Heiser, N.A., Turner, S.M., Beidel, D.C., and Roberson-Nay, R. (2009). Differentiating Social Phobia from Shyness. *Journal of Anxiety Disorders*, 23: 469–476.

Hirsch, C.R., Clark, D.M., Mathews, A., and Williams, R. (2003). Self-images Play a Causal Role in Social Phobia. *Behaviour Research and Therapy*, 41: 909–921.

Lieb, R., Wittchen, H.-U., Höfler, M., Fuetsch, M., Stein, M.B., and Merikangas, K.R. (2000). Parental Psychopathology, Parenting Styles, and the Risk of Social Phobia in Offspring. *Archives of General Psychiatry*, 57: 859–866.

Maner, J.K., Miller, S.L., Schmidt, N.B., and Eckel, L.A. (2008). Submitting to Defeat: Social Anxiety, Dominance Threat, and Decrements in Testosterone. *Psychological Science*, 19: 764–768.

Mosing, M.A., Gordon, S.D., Medland, S.E., Statham, D.J., Nelson, E.C., Heath, A.C., Martin, N.G., and Wray, N.R. (2009). Genetic and Environmental Influences on the Co-morbidity between Depression, Panic Disorder, Agoraphobia, and Social Phobia: A Twin Study. *Depression and Anxiety*, 26: 1004–1011.

Siqueland, L., Kendall, P.C., and Steinberg, L. (1996). Anxiety in Children: Perceived Family Environments and Observed Family Interaction. *Journal of Clinical Child and Adolescent Psychology*, 25: 225–237.

Stein, D.J. (2009). Social Anxiety Disorder in the West and in the East. *Annals of Clinical Psychiatry*, 21: 109–117.

Wells, A. (1997). *Cognitive Therapy of Anxiety Disorders: A Practice Manual and Conceptual Guide* (Chichester: John Wiley).

Wild, J., Clark, D.M., Ehlers, A., and McManus, F. (2008). Perception of Arousal in Social Anxiety: Effects of False Feedback During a Social Interaction. *Journal of Behavior Therapy and Experimental Psychiatry*, 39: 102–116.

Chapter 7

American Psychiatric Association. (2000). *Diagnostic and Statistical Manual of Mental Disorders*, 4th edn., Text Revision. (Arlington, VA: American Psychiatric Association).

Barloon, T.J. and Noyes, R., Jr. (1997). Charles Darwin and Panic Disorder. *Journal of the American Medical Association*, 277: 138–141.

Barlow, D.H. (2002). *Anxiety and its Disorders*, 2nd edn. (New York: Guilford Press).

Clark, D.M. and Fairburn, C.G. (eds). *Science and Practice of Cognitive Behaviour Therapy*. (Oxford and New York: Oxford University Press).

Craske, M.G., Lang, A.J., Mystkowski, J.L., Zucker, B.G., Bystritsky, A., and Yan-Go, F. (2002). Does Nocturnal Panic Represent a More

Severe Form of Panic Disorder? *Journal of Nervous and Mental Disease*, 190: 611–618.

Ehlers, A. (1993). Somatic Symptoms and Panic Attacks: A Retrospective Study of Learning Experiences. *Behaviour Research and Therapy*, 31: 269–278.

Ehlers, A. and Breuer, P. (1992). Increased Cardiac Awareness in Panic Disorder. *Journal of Abnormal Psychology*, 101: 371–382.

Eley, T.C., Stirling, L., Ehlers, A., Gregory, A.M., and Clark, D.M. (2004). Heart-beat Perception, Panic/Somatic Symptoms and Anxiety Sensitivity in Children. *Behaviour Research and Therapy*, 42: 439–448.

Goodwin, R.D., Fergusson, D.M., and Horwood, L.J. (2005). Childhood Abuse and Familial Violence and the Risk of Panic Attacks and Panic Disorder in Young Adulthood. *Psychological Medicine*, 35: 881–890.

Kessler, R.C., Chiu, W.T., Jin, R., Ruscio, A.M., Shear, K., and Walters, E.E. (2006). The Epidemiology of Panic Attacks, Panic Disorder, and Agoraphobia in the National Comorbidity Survey Replication. *Archives of General Psychiatry*, 63: 415–424.

Klein, D.F. (1993). False Suffocation Alarms, Spontaneous Panics, and Related Conditions: An Integrative Hypothesis. *Archives of General Psychiatry*, 50: 306–317.

Lau, J.Y.F., Gregory, A.M., Goldwin, M.A., Pine, D.S., and Eley, T.C. (2007). Assessing Gene–Environment Interactions on Anxiety Symptom Subtypes Across Childhood and Adolescence. *Development and Psychopathology*, 19: 1129–1146.

Plomin, R., DeFries, J.C., McClearn, G.E., and McGuffin, P. (2008). *Behavioral Genetics*, 5th edn. (New York: Worth).

Rachman, S. (2004). *Anxiety*, 2nd edn. (Hove and New York: Psychology Press).

Rapee, R., Mattick, R., and Murrell, E. (1986). Cognitive Mediation in the Affective Component of Spontaneous Panic Attacks. *Journal of Behavior Therapy and Experimental Psychiatry*, 17: 245–253.

Salkovskis, P.M., Clark, D.M., Hackmann, A., Wells, A., and Gelder, M.G. (1999). An Experimental Investigation of the Role of Safety-seeking Behaviours in the Maintenance of Panic Disorder with Agoraphobia. *Behaviour Research and Therapy*, 37: 559–574.

Schmidt, N.B., Lerew, D.R., and Jackson, R.J. (1997). The Role of Anxiety Sensitivity in the Pathogenesis of Panic: Prospective Evaluation of Spontaneous Panic Attacks During Acute Stress. *Journal of Abnormal Psychology*, 106: 355–364.

Smoller, J.W., Block, S.R., and Young, M.M. (2009). Genetics of Anxiety Disorders: The Complex Road from DSM to DNA. *Depression and Anxiety*, 26: 965–975.

Chapter 8

American Psychiatric Association. (2000). *Diagnostic and Statistical Manual of Mental Disorders*, 4th edn., Text Revision. (Arlington, VA: American Psychiatric Association).

Barlow, D.H. (2002). *Anxiety and its Disorders*, 2nd edn. (New York: Guilford Press).

Borkovec, T.D., Ray, W.J., and Stöber, J. (1998). Worry: A Cognitive Phenomenon Intimately Linked to Affective, Physiological, and Interpersonal Behavioral Processes. *Cognitive Therapy and Research*, 22: 561–576.

Davey, G.C.L. and Wells, A. (eds.) (2006). *Worry and its Psychological Disorders: Theory, Assessment and Treatment*. (Chichester: John Wiley).

Kendler, K.S., Gardner, C.O., Gatz, M., and Pedersen, N.L. (2007). The Sources of Co-morbidity Between Major Depression and Generalized Anxiety Disorder in a Swedish National Twin Sample. *Psychological Medicine*, 37: 453–462.

Meyer, T.J., Miller, M.L., Metzger, R.L., and Borkovec, T.D. (1990). Development and Validation of the Penn State Worry Questionnaire. *Behaviour Research and Therapy*, 28: 487–495.

Moffitt, T.E., Caspi, A., Harrington, H., Milne, B.J., Melchior, M., Goldberg, D., and Poulton, R. (2007). Generalized Anxiety Disorder and Depression: Childhood Risk Factors in a Birth Cohort Followed to Age 32. *Psychological Medicine*, 37: 441–452.

Muris, P., Meesters, C., Merckelbach, H., Hülsenbeck, P. (2000). Worry in Children is Related to Perceived Parental Rearing and Attachment. *Behaviour Research and Therapy*, 38: 487–497.

Paulesu, E., Sambugaro, E., Torti, T., Danelli, L., Ferri, F., Scialfa, G., Sberna, M., Ruggiero, G.M., Bottini, G., and Sassaroli, S. (2010). Neural Correlates of Worry in Generalized Anxiety Disorder and in Normal Controls: A Functional MRI Study. *Psychological Medicine*, 40: 117–124.

Peasley-Miklus, D. and Vrana, S.R. (2000). Effect of Worrisome and Relaxing Thinking on Fearful Emotional Processing. *Behaviour Research and Therapy*, 38: 129–144.

Plomin, R., DeFries, J.C., McClearn, G.E., and McGuffin, P. (2008). *Behavioral Genetics*, 5th edn. (New York: Worth).

Rachman, S. (2004). *Anxiety*, 2nd edn. (Hove and New York: Psychology Press).

Tallis, F., Davey, G. and Capuzzo, N. (1994). The Phenomenology of Non-Pathological Worry: A Preliminary Investigation. In G. Davey and F. Tallis (eds.) *Worrying: Perspectives on Theory, Assessment and Treatment*. (Chichester: Wiley)

Vasey, M.W. and Borkovec, T.D. (1992). A Catastrophizing Assessment of Worrisome Thoughts. *Cognitive Therapy and Research*, 16: 505–520.

Chapter 9

Abramowitz, J.S., Wheaton, M.G., and Storch, E.A. (2008). The Status of Hoarding as a Symptom of Obsessive-Compulsive Disorder. *Behaviour Research and Therapy*, 46: 1026–1033.

Abramowitz, J.S., Taylor, S., and McKay, D. (2009). Obsessive-Compulsive Disorder. *Lancet*, 374: 491–499.

American Psychiatric Association. (2000). *Diagnostic and Statistical Manual of Mental Disorders*, 4th edn., Text Revision. (Arlington, VA: American Psychiatric Association).

Barlow, D.H. (2002). *Anxiety and its Disorders*, 2nd edn. (New York: Guilford Press).

Berrios, G. and Porter, R. (eds.) (1995). *A History of Clinical Psychiatry: The Origin and History of Psychiatric Disorders*. (London: Athlone Press).

Briggs, E.S. and Price, I.R. (2009). The Relationship between Adverse Childhood Experience and Obsessive-Compulsive Symptoms and Beliefs: The Role of Anxiety, Depression, and Experiential Avoidance. *Journal of Anxiety Disorders*, 23: 1037–1046.

Cath, D.C., van Grootheest, D.S., Willemsen, G., van Oppen, P., and Boomsma, D.I. (2008). Environmental Factors in Obsessive-Compulsive Behavior: Evidence from Discordant and Concordant Monozygotic Twins. *Behavior Genetics*, 38: 108–120.

Dougherty, D.D., Baer, L., Cosgrove, G.R., Cassem, E.H., Price, B.H., Nierenberg, A.A., Jenike, M.A., and Rauch, S.L. (2002). Prospective Long-Term Follow-Up of 44 Patients who Received Cingulotomy for Treatment-Refractory Obsessive-Compulsive Disorder. *American Journal of Psychiatry*, 159: 269–275.

Klinger, E. (1978). Modes of Normal Conscious Flow. In K. S. Pope and J. L. Singer (eds.), *The Stream of Consciousness*. (New York: Plenum Press).

Klinger, E. (1996). The Contents of Thoughts: Interference as the Downside of Adaptive Normal Mechanisms in Thought Flow. In I. G. Sarason, G. R. Pierce, and B. R. Sarason (eds.), *Cognitive Interference: Theories, Methods, and Findings*. (Mahwah, NJ: Lawrence Erlbaum Associates).

Mataix-Cols, D., Wooderson, S., Lawrence, N., Brammer, M.J., Speckens, A., and Phillips, M.L. (2004). Distinct Neural Correlates of Washing, Checking, and Hoarding Symptom Dimensions in Obsessive-Compulsive Disorder. *Archives of General Psychiatry*, 61: 564–576.

Miller, C.H. and Hedges, D.W. (2008). Scrupulosity Disorder: An Overview and Introductory Analysis. *Journal of Anxiety Disorders*, 22: 1042–1058.

Plomin, R., DeFries, J.C., McClearn, G.E., and McGuffin, P. (2008). *Behavioral Genetics*, 5th edn. (New York: Worth).

Rachman, S. (2004). *Anxiety*, 2nd edn. (Hove and New York: Psychology Press).

Rachman, S. and de Silva, P. (1978). Abnormal and Normal Obsessions. *Behaviour Research and Therapy*, 16: 233–248.

Ruscio, A.M., Stein, D.J., Chiu, W.T., and Kessler, R.C. (2010). The Epidemiology of Obsessive-Compulsive Disorder in the National Comorbidity Replication Survey. *Molecular Psychiatry*, 15: 53–63.

Salkovskis, P.M. (1999). Understanding and Treating Obsessive-Compulsive Disorder. *Behaviour Research and Therapy*, 37: S29–S52.

Tolin, D.F., Abramowitz, J.S., Przeworski, A., and Foa, E.B. (2002). Thought Suppression in Obsessive-Compulsive Disorder. *Behaviour Research and Therapy*, 40: 1255–1274.

van den Hout, M.A., Engelhard, I.M., de Boer, C., du Bois, A., and Dek, E. (2008). Perseverative and Compulsive-like Staring Causes Uncertainty About Perception. *Behaviour Research and Therapy*, 46: 1300–1304.

van den Hout, M.A. and Kindt, M. (2003). Repeated Checking Causes Memory Distrust. *Behaviour Research and Therapy*, 41: 301–316.

van Grootheest, D.S., Boomsma, D.I., Hettema, J.M., and Kendler, K.S. (2007). Heritability of Obsessive-Compulsive Symptom Dimensions. *American Journal of Medical Genetics*, 147B: 473–478.

Afifi, T.O., Asmundson, G.J.G., Taylor, S., and Jang, K.L. (2010). The Role of Genes and Environment on Trauma Exposure and Posttraumatic Stress Disorder Symptoms: A Review of Twin Studies. *Clinical Psychology Review*, 30: 101–112.

American Psychiatric Association. (2000). *Diagnostic and Statistical Manual of Mental Disorders*, 4th edn., Text Revision. (Arlington, VA: American Psychiatric Association).

Asmundson, J.G.J., Stapleton, J.A., and Taylor, S. (2004). Are Avoidance and Numbing Distinct PTSD Symptom Clusters? *Journal of Traumatic Stress*, 17: 467–475.

Barlow, D.H. (2002). *Anxiety and its Disorders*, 2nd edn. (New York: Guilford Press).

Berrios, G. and Porter, R. (eds.) (1995). *A History of Clinical Psychiatry: The Origin and History of Psychiatric Disorders.* (London: Athlone Press).

Brewin, C.R., Dalgleish, T., and Joseph, S. (1996). A Dual Representation Theory of Posttraumatic Stress Disorder. *Psychological Review*, 103: 670–686.

Cohen Silver, R., Holman, E.A., McIntosh, D.N., Poulin, M., Gil-Rivas, V., and Pizarro, J. (2006). Coping with a National Trauma: A Nationwide Longitudinal Study of Responses to the Terrorist Attacks of September 11. In Y. Neria, R. Gross, R. Marshall, and E. Susser (eds.), *9/11: Mental Health in the Wake of Terrorist Attacks*. (Cambridge: Cambridge University Press).

Cox, B.J., Mota, N., Clara, I., and Asmundson, G.J.G. (2008). The Symptom Structure of Posttraumatic Stress Disorder in the National Comorbidity Replication Survey. *Journal of Anxiety Disorders*, 22: 1523–1528.

DeLisi, L.E. (2005). The New York Experience: Terrorist Attacks on September 11, 2001. In J.J. López-Ibor, G. Christodoulou, M. Maj, N. Sartorius, and A. Okasha (eds.), *Disasters and Mental Health*. (Chichester: John Wiley).

Ehlers, A. and Clark, D.M. (2000). A Cognitive Model of Posttraumatic Stress Disorder. *Behaviour Research and Therapy*, 38: 319–345.

Ehring, T., Ehlers, A., and Glucksman, E. (2008). Do Cognitive Models Help in Predicting the Severity of Posttraumatic Stress Disorder, Phobia, and Depression after Motor Vehicle Accidents?

A Prospective Longitudinal Study. *Journal of Consulting and Clinical Psychology*, 76: 219–230.

de Jong, J.T.V.M., Komproe, I.H., van Ommeren, M., El Masri, M., Araya, M., Khaled, N., van de Put, W., and Somasundaram, D. (2001). Lifetime Events and Posttraumatic Stress Disorder in 4 Postconflict Settings. *Journal of the American Medical Association*, 286: 555–562.

Kessler, R.C., Sonnega, A., Bromet, E., Hughes, M., and Nelson, C.B. (1995). Posttraumatic Stress Disorder in the National Comorbidity Survey. *Archives of General Psychiatry*, 52: 1048–1060.

Mol, S.S.L., Arntz, A., Metsemakers, J.F.M., Dinant, G.J., Vilters-Van Montfort, P.A.P., and Knottnerus, J.A. (2005). Symptoms of Post-Traumatic Stress Disorder After Non-Traumatic Events: Evidence from an Open Population Study. *British Journal of Psychiatry*, 186: 494–499.

Rachman, S. (2004). *Anxiety*, 2nd edn. (Hove and New York: Psychology Press).

Reyes, G., Elhai, J.D., and Ford, J.D. (eds.) (2008). *The Encyclopedia of Psychological Trauma*. (Hoboken, NJ: John Wiley).

Stein, M.B., Jang, K.L., Taylor, S., Vernon, P.A., and Livesley, W.J. (2002). Genetic and Environmental Influences on Trauma Exposure and Posttraumatic Stress Disorder Symptoms: A Twin Study. *American Journal of Psychiatry*, 159: 1675–1681.

Wang, Z., Neylan, T.C., Mueller, S.G., Lenoci, M., Truran, D., Marmar, C.R., Weiner, M.W., and Schuff, N. (2010). Magnetic Resonance Imaging of Hippocampal Subfields in Posttraumatic Stress Disorder. *Archives of General Psychiatry*, 67: 296–303.

Whalley, M.G. and Brewin, C.R. (2007). Mental Health Following Terrorist Attacks. *British Journal of Psychiatry*, 190: 94–96.

Chapter 11

Blank, L., Grimsley, M., Goyder, E., Ellis, E., and Peters, J. (2007). Community-Based Lifestyle Interventions: Changing Behaviour and Improving Health. *Journal of Public Health*, 29: 236–245.

Gelder, M., Harrison, P., and Cowen, P. (2006). *Shorter Oxford Textbook of Psychiatry*. (Oxford: Oxford University Press).

Gerrardi, M., Rothbaum, B.O., Ressler, K., Heekin, M., and Rizzo, A. (2008). Virtual Reality Exposure Therapy Using a Virtual Iraq: Case Report. *Journal of Traumatic Stress*, 21: 209–213.

Grey, N. (ed.) (2009). *A Casebook of Cognitive Therapy for Traumatic Stress Reactions.* (Hove: Routledge).

Grossman, P., Niemann, L., Schmidt, S., and Walach, H. (2004). Mindfulness-Based Stress Reduction and Health Benefits: A Meta-Analysis. *Journal of Psychosomatic Research,* 57: 35–43.

Healy, D. (2009). *Psychiatric Drugs Explained,* 5th edn. (Oxford: Elsevier).

Kirkwood, G., Rampes, H., Tuffrey, V., Richardson, J., and Pilkington, K. (2005). Yoga for Anxiety: A Systematic Review of the Research. *British Journal of Sports Medicine,* 39: 884–891.

Manzoni, G.M., Pagnini, F., Castelnuovo, G., and Molinari, E. (2008). Relaxation Training for Anxiety: A Ten-Years Systematic Review with Meta-Analysis. *BMC Psychiatry,* 8: 41.

McManus, S., Meltzer, H., Brugha, T., Bebbington, P., and Jenkins, R. (2009). *Adult Psychiatric Morbidity in England, 2007.* (Leeds: NHS Information Centre).

Moyer, C.A., Rounds, J., and Hannum, J.W. (2004). A Meta-Analysis of Massage Therapy Research. *Psychological Bulletin,* 130: 3–18.

National Institute for Health and Clinical Excellence (2005). *Post-Traumatic Stress Disorder* (London: NICE).

National Institute for Health and Clinical Excellence (2005). *Obsessive-Compulsive Disorder* (London: NICE).

National Institute for Health and Clinical Excellence (2007). *Anxiety (Amended)* (London: NICE).

NHS Primary Care Guidelines (2004). *Phobic Disorders* (World Health Organization).

Öst, L.G. (1997). Rapid Treatment of Specific Phobias. In G.C.L. Davey (ed.), *Phobias: A Handbook of Theory, Research and Treatment.* (Chichester: Wiley).

Otto, M.W., Behar, E., Smits, J.A.J., and Hofmann, S.G. (2009). Combining Pharmacological and Cognitive Behavioral Therapy in the Treatment of Anxiety Disorders. In M.M. Antony and M.B. Stein (eds.), *Oxford Handbook of Anxiety and Related Disorders.* (Oxford and New York: Oxford University Press).

Powers, M.B. and Emmelkamp, P.M.G. (2008). Virtual Reality Exposure Therapy for Anxiety Disorders: A Meta-Analysis. *Journal of Anxiety Disorders,* 22: 561–569.

Salmon, P. (2001). Effects of Physical Exercise on Anxiety, Depression, and Sensitivity to Stress: A Unifying Theory. *Clinical Psychology Review,* 21: 33–61.

Schulz, K.F., Altman, D.G., and Moher, D. (2010). CONSORT 2010 Statement: Updated Guidelines for Reporting Parallel Group Randomized Trials. *Annals of Internal Medicine*, 152: 1–8.

Walker, J.R., Vincent, N., and Furer, P. (2009). Self-Help Treatments for Anxiety Disorders. In M.M. Antony and M.B. Stein (eds.), *Oxford Handbook of Anxiety and Related Disorders*. (Oxford and New York: Oxford University Press).

Weiss, D. S., and Marmar, C. R. (1997). The Impact of Event Scale–Revised. In J. Wilson & T. M. Keane (eds.), *Assessing Psychological Trauma and PTSD*. (New York: Guilford).

Further reading

If you'd like more information about anxiety disorders in general, we've devoted a substantial section to them in *Know Your Mind: Everyday Emotional and Psychological Problems and How to Overcome Them* (Rodale, 2009). Also worth checking out is Helen Kennerley's *Overcoming Anxiety* (Robinson, 2009).

On the Internet, see www.anxietyuk.org.uk, the website of the charity Anxiety UK, and www.adaa.org, which is run by the Anxiety Disorders Association of America.

Phobias

Edmund Bourne, *The Anxiety and Phobia Workbook*, 5th edn. (New Harbinger, 2011)
Warren Mansell, *Coping with Fears and Phobias* (Oneworld, 2007)
http://topuk.org (Triumph Over Phobia UK)

Shyness and social phobia

Gillian Butler, *Overcoming Social Anxiety and Shyness* (Robinson, 2009)
Murray Stein and John Walker, *Triumph Over Shyness* (Anxiety Disorders Association of America, 2002)
www.anxietynetwork.com
www.social-anxiety.org.uk
www.socialphobia.org

Panic disorder

Stanley Rachman and Padmal de Silva, *Panic Disorder: The Facts* (Oxford University Press, 2009)

Derrick Silove and Vijaya Manicavasagar, *Overcoming Panic and Agoraphobia* (Robinson, 2009)

http://www.nomorepanic.co.uk

http://nopanic.org.uk

http://anxietypanic.com

Worry and generalized anxiety disorder

Robert Leahy, *The Worry Cure* (New Harbinger, 2006)

Kevin Meares and Mark Freeston, *Overcoming Worry* (Robinson, 2008)

Obsessive-compulsive disorder

Christine Purdon and David Clark, *Overcoming Obsessive Thoughts* (New Harbinger, 2005)

Padmal de Silva and Stanley Rachman, *Obsessive-Compulsive Disorder* (Oxford University Press, 2009)

David Veale and Rob Willson, *Overcoming Obsessive-Compulsive Disorder* (Robinson, 2009)

http://www.ocdaction.org.uk

http://www.ocfoundation.org

Post-traumatic stress disorder

Barbara Olasov Rothbaum, Edna Foa, and Elizabeth Hembree, *Reclaiming Your Life from a Traumatic Experience* (Oxford University Press, 2007)

Glenn Schiraldi, *The Post-Traumatic Stress Disorder Sourcebook*, 2nd edn. (McGraw-Hill, 2009)

http://www.ptsd.va.gov

Index

Expand your collection of
VERY SHORT INTRODUCTIONS

AUTISM
A Very Short Introduction
Uta Frith

This *Very Short Introduction* offers a clear statement on what is currently known about autism and Asperger syndrome. Explaining the vast array of different conditions that hide behind these two labels, and looking at symptoms from the full spectrum of autistic disorders, it explores the possible causes for the apparent rise in autism and also evaluates the links with neuroscience, psychology, brain development, genetics, and environmental causes including MMR and Thimerosal. This short, authoritative, and accessible book also explores the psychology behind social impairment and savantism and sheds light on what it is like to live inside the mind of the sufferer.

www.oup.com/vsi

PSYCHOLOGY
A Very Short Introduction
Gillian Butler and Freda McManus

Psychology: A Very Short Introduction provides an up-to-date overview of the main areas of psychology, translating complex psychological matters, such as perception, into readable topics so as to make psychology accessible for newcomers to the subject. The authors use everyday examples as well as research findings to foster curiosity about how and why the mind works in the way it does, and why we behave in the ways we do. This book explains why knowing about psychology is important and relevant to the modern world.

'a very readable, stimulating, and well-written introduction to psychology which combines factual information with a welcome honesty about the current limits of knowledge. It brings alive the fascination and appeal of psychology, its significance and implications, and its inherent challenges.'

Anthony Clare

'This excellent text provides a succinct account of how modern psychologists approach the study of the mind and human behaviour. ... the best available introduction to the subject.'

Anthony Storr